Goodbye Insomnia,
Hello Sleep

Goodbye Insomnia, Hello Sleep

Samuel Dunkell, M.D.

A BIRCH LANE PRESS BOOK
Published by Carol Publishing Group

To Nicholas and Jennifer Jenkins
Sleepers of the new age
(See chapter 13)

A Birch Lane Press Book
Published by Carol Publishing Group
Birch Lane Press is a registered trademark of Carol Communications, Inc.
Editorial Offices: 600 Madison Avenue, New York, N.Y. 10022
Sales and Distribution Offices: 120 Enterprise Avenue, Secaucus, N.J. 07094
In Canada: Canadian Manda Group, P.O. Box 920, Station U, Toronto, Ontario M8Z 5P9
Queries regarding rights and permissions should be addressed to Carol Publishing Group,
600 Madison Avenue, New York, N.Y. 10022

Carol Publishing Group books are available at special discounts for bulk purchases, sales
promotion, fund-raising, or educational purposes. Special editions can be created to
specifications. For details, contact: Special Sales Department, Carol Publishing Group,
120 Enterprise Avenue, Secaucus, N.J. 07094

Manufactured in the United States of America
10 9 8 7 6 5 4 3 2 1

Library of Congress Cataloging-in-Publication Data
Dunkell, Samuel.
Goodbye insomnia, hello sleep / by Samuel Dunkell.
p.   cm.
"A Birch Lane Press book".
ISBN 1-55972-247-9
1. Insomnia—Popular works.   I. Title.
RC548.D86   1994
616.8'498—dc20   94-18114
CIP

Contents

Preface

The answering machine at Insomnia Medical Services held a number of messages that were left for me in the early morning hours. A popular national magazine had carried a story on insomnia in which I was quoted. The early dawn callers had apparently just survived another sleepless night. The voices were low, halting, and slurred—an effect caused, I assume, either by total exhaustion or by sleeping pills that hadn't worked. The tone was uniformly resigned and hopeless, with a barely concealed anger that seemed to ask, "Why can't I sleep? Why can't I seem to do anything about it? How much longer must I endure this?"

Who are these callers? Are they just a few poor souls who unluckily had a run of sleepless nights befall them out of the blue?

If, like these callers, you suffer from the plague of sleep loss—whether for a few occasional nights or, as in the case of some of my patients, for decades—you are not alone. Repeated surveys in the United States and overseas have shown that insomnia afflicts fully one-third of the population and that half of its sufferers have experienced enough distress and disability to seek professional help.

Until recently, though, if you had a serious sleep difficulty not too much could have been done that really would have helped you, especially if you had chronic insomnia. Although nostrums and practices to relieve sleeplessness go back to the cave dwellers, no universally effective solution had been found that relieved long lasting sleeplessness completely and reliably.

However, sleep sufferers, do not despair. The picture has changed. The last few decades have seen the emergence of a new

scientific discipline—sleep medicine. The result of this development has been the application of a surge of new discoveries about
sleep. Does this benefit you directly? Will it help you recover your
refreshing sleep of the past? The answer is definitely yes. I find
that virtually everyone who comes to consult me about a sleep
problem is helped.

It was during my psychiatric residency that I initially became
aware of the newly developing field of sleep medicine. Space was
exceedingly scarce in the section of the hospital where I worked.
I sometimes saw my patients in a room that was set aside for sleep
research at night and left free during the day, except for occasional
use as a makeshift office. The setting was weird. The couches and
most of the furniture in this room were bedecked with white sheets
during the day, leaving only the large carbon-encrusted drumrolls,
then employed to record sleep events, as dark presences in a silent
world.

Perhaps it was the memory of the intriguing quality of this room
that, in the late 1960s, led me to read one of the early collections
of research on sleep. The material became quite addictive. I was
increasingly fascinated by the stream of sleep research literature,
which at that time was relatively small, and watched as the early
trickle became a wave of enlightening and useful knowledge.

In retrospect, it was probably this focus on the unfolding events
of sleep research, combined with the constant sight of patients
lying before me on the couch, that crystallized my initial insight
that we prefer sleeping positions which reflect our intrinsic personalities and stances in life. I was particularly impressed by the
reliance sleepers had on these positions to enable them to fall
asleep and remain asleep.

Since sleeplessness has always been an early warning sign of
disturbance in my patients' lives, the symptom of insomnia became
an important clinical phenomenon to be explored.

I approach insomnia, in this book, from a broad perspective. In
addition to the early sections describing the essential facts about
insomnia and describing the ways to successfully identify and overcome your sleep difficulty, later portions explore other important
topics: the special sleep problems of the child, adolescent, and
senior populations; sleeping pill use; sleep hygiene—ways to cul-
tivate good sleep habits and eliminate sleep disruptive practices;
and using workable relaxation techniques to help you fall asleep
easily.

Other chapters deal with aspects of the sleep experience that expand our understanding of the unique nature of the whole sleep world. For example, I look at dreams not only for their meanings, but also in terms of what we can discover about insomnia from them; and in another chapter I present discoveries and findings of my own in the areas of sleep and insomnia that have never before been published.

In the final chapter I examine the connections between day fitness and sleep fitness.

If you practice fitness during the day and cannot sleep at night, then your fitness program is like the sound of one hand clapping; your pursuit of fitness by day is compromised by your sleep difficulties at night.

If you are in the estimated eighty-five percent of chronic insomniacs who are doing nothing about their unending sleeplessness, you should become aware of the many recent advances in sleep medicine. It is unfortunate, since these developments—behavior therapies for insomnia, the development of bright light therapy and short term psychotherapy–counseling treatment methods, the widespread growth of clinics devoted to insomnia and the increase in sleep centers, the proposal to establish a National Institute of Health for sleep, the effective use of instrumentation for recording and measuring sleep events (like all-night EEG recording and objective tests for daytime sleepiness), the extensive growth of knowledge about sleep disorders, and many more advances and breakthroughs—have put us in a position to make the myth of helplessness about insomnia truly archaic.

You are welcomed to the pages of this book to find out about these remarkable achievements and how they can be applied to overcome your own sleep problems. Learn to be a sleep winner and not a sleep loser.

In the chapters that follow I will show how your insomnia can be vanquished. We have the ability to pinpoint the causes of sleep loss and the specific techniques to deal with the types and patterns in which they beset you. The promise of the title is no illusion. The means for undoing the discomforting and debilitating effects of your insomnia are now at hand.

To find your own path to recovery, *Read this and sleep*!

In the summer of 1989, an archeologist digging in the ancient city of Nimrud, once the military capital of the Assyrian kingdom, uncovered a stone chamber that was presumed to be the tomb of the daughter and granddaughter of Sargon, the ruler of this 8th century B.C. empire. The cuneiform script on the wall was deciphered and discovered to be a curse on anyone who opened the tomb, and read "If anyone lays his hands on my tomb and opens my grave, I pray to the gods of the nether world that his soul shall roam in the scorching sun after death. . . . Let the ghost of insomnia take hold of him for ever and ever."

New York Times, Science Watch
August 15, 1989

Archeologists, however, do not need to feel inhibited by fear of eternal haunting by the ghost of insomnia. Insomnia is no longer the curse it has been. Our current research and clinical knowledge and the new ways to evaluate, diagnose, and treat insomnia have finally defused this damnation, as the following chapters will make clear.

Goodbye Insomnia,
Hello Sleep

Chapter 1

The Night Life of the Insomniac

Short Sleep, Long Sleep, Average Sleep

How much sleep does the average adult need? There is no absolute best amount of sleep, just as there is no best height or weight.

I sometimes get calls from persons who tell me that they sleep only five or six hours a night, and anxiously ask if this means that they have insomnia. When I ask them how they feel and function during the day, their usual response is, "Quite well." Hearing this, I tell them that they are short sleepers, not insomniacs, and to continue their good sleep, unperturbed. They are merely troubled by the fact that they do not live up to the myth of the fixed necessity for eight hours of sleep. Very likely these callers slept less than others did as young children and have a biologically built-in short sleep need.

Short sleepers get six hours or less sleep time a night. Some even sleep as little as three or four hours but, like prizefighters in the first round, awaken bright eyed and alert, eager to do battle. Their sleep time may be short, but it is also efficient. They awaken less often during the night, and sleep deeply—dallying less in the lighter stages of sleep. Short sleepers have energetic, driving, chipper personalities, and are highly practical—firmly anchored in the concrete details and goals of their everyday lives. They don't even seem to have time to dream. If they do, their dreams are few in number, short, and mundane, and their dream recall is sparse. The condensed sleep of short sleepers shows that it is the quality of sleep, not just the quantity, that counts!

Some busy individuals even train themselves to become short

sleepers in order to wring as much productivity out of their days as possible. President Lyndon Johnson often slept only four hours a night, but also took catnaps during the day. The 1972 Democratic nominee, George McGovern, used to astound reporters traveling with him by his ability to take twenty minute naps, effortlessly falling asleep in the midst of the chaos of his campaign plane.

Long sleepers, by contrast, sleep nine hours or more each night and may even need as many as ten or twelve hours in order to feel refreshed and to function well the next day. Long sleepers tend to be introspective and ambivalent in their approach to life. Perhaps, like Rip Van Winkle, they linger too long in the underworld of sleep, awakening belatedly to a bewildering universe. They dream more than most people, and their dreams are longer and more complex, with lavish dream recall. Although they are also prone to depression and other emotional problems, they are usually creative types and inclined to deal with abstraction.

The majority of us are variable sleepers, able to adjust the length of our sleep according to our fatigue and the needs of the moment.

Geography and climate may play a role in sleep length. Southerners and Westerners need more sleep than do people from other areas! Why? An explanation that has been offered is that their towns and highways are not as congested as those in the rest of the country, giving them the luxury of sleeping later before having to hustle off to work.

Overall, the sleep lengths of the population range from four to ten hours per night. Most adults sleep between seven and a half and eight and a half hours. Ten percent sleep nine or more hours and five percent sleep fewer than six hours.

Our individual sleep needs are set by inborn tendencies, training, and personal styles, as well as by the constraints of our schedules. As a rule, we go to bed when we want to, but get up when we have to. This practice can lead to a sleep debt that accumulates during the work week and is made up by us on weekends, when there is a tendency to sleep later.

Who Are Normal Sleepers?

Normal sleepers are satisfied sleepers who wake up refreshed and have no complaints about their ability to sleep. They have regular sleep habits, fall asleep and awaken at roughly the same times, and rarely find it necessary either to force sleep or to fight it off. Their sleep is a nightly rest cure.

If you are puzzled about how much sleep you actually need, there is a simple way to estimate the amount. Go to bed at the same time every night and see when you get up without using an alarm. This is best done over a two week period, perhaps on vacation when there are no work demands. Use the first week to overcome any outstanding sleep debt, and during the second, note the figures for each night, and then average your nightly sleep need. Remember, there is no absolute best sleep amount for everyone!

Pseudo-Insomniacs

There is another group of sleepers who complain of fatigue and poor sleep, yet show no detectable objective signs of insomnia in sleep laboratory examination, despite their complaints. Sleep researchers are torn about this group. Are they "Pseudo-insomniacs," or do they really have a valid complaint? When given treatment, they do report subjective sleep improvement, but this may be a matter of their "convincing themselves" of a change. Some authorities believe that they are like the princess who slept on a hundred mattresses and still felt the pea. Are these sleepers, in fact, more sensitive to brief awakenings, position changes, and dreaming than other sleepers?

Nighttime Awakenings

Although it may not be easily recalled, everyone wakes occasionally during the night. We don't remember because memory is affected during sleep. Events that take place immediately prior to sleep are often forgotten. It takes seven or more minutes of steady wake time for a memory—like a photograph in a developing solution—to be fixated sufficiently for recall. That's why it is difficult to underline the precise moment we fall asleep, or why we forget phone calls that occur in the middle of the night, or what was said during the call if it was brief.

The number and duration of nighttime awakenings vary with age. The typical young adult awakens twice, with the number of awakenings increasing steadily after the age of forty. The average

amount of time spent awake during a wake period in early adulthood is approximately two minutes, increasing to five minutes in
later life.

What Is Insomnia? Who Gets It? What Causes It?

The portrait painted so far has been that of the normal sleeper,
allowing for accepted variations between short and long sleepers.
When it comes to insomniacs—or "insom-maniacs," as the hu-
morist Richard Armour described himself and fellow sufferers—
the picture changes considerably. Research has shown that poor
sleepers have a greater than average number of brief (or even long)
wakes during the night; they are restless and have more frequent
shiftings in and out of different sleep stages, spending more time
in the lighter, less refreshing stages.

The two major objective criteria used to define insomnia are:
sleep onset latency (the length of time it takes to fall asleep initially), and sleep efficiency (the proportion of time actually spent
asleep during the night in relation to the total time spent in bed).
If falling asleep takes forty-five minutes or longer, it is seen, by
convention, as indicative of the presence of insomnia. Insomnia is
also present if less than eighty-five percent of the time in bed is
spent sleeping.

The typical insomniac, mired in sleep loss fatigue, is aware that
his daytime symptoms are crucial. Though distressed by the night's
struggles, the primary concern of the insomniac is how he or she
feels during the day. If there are no symptoms of fatigue, sleepiness, irritability, diminished job performance, and poor concentration the following day, there is no insomnia! Many of the typical
daytime symptoms can be tested objectively and used to evaluate
the quality of a night's sleep.

Transient Insomnia results from an acute situational stress and
lasts only a few days, disappearing when the stress lets up.

In Short Term Insomnia, the sleeplessness has a longer duration,
extending from a few weeks to three or four months.

When insomnia lasts more than four months it becomes Chronic
Insomnia, the major concern of this book.

It is incorrect to rely only on the worst nights of sleeplessness in
evaluating insomnia. The entire, long-range, general pattern should
be examined. Temporary sleep loss is not insomnia. Insomnia oc-

curs when sleep loss lasts at least half the nights of a week over a span of several weeks.

Semantics enter into definitions of insomnia. People who were asked if they had insomnia replied "yes" in only twenty percent of the cases in a population survey. On the other hand, when they were asked if they had difficulty in sleeping, one-third of the population answered in the affirmative.

What the Sleepless Do at Night

Insomniacs leave the bed frequently, try to sleep in another room, or go into the living room. Thirty-eight percent watch TV or read. Others do crossword puzzles, go to the kitchen and raid the refrigerator, do housework to tire themselves out, do bills, take baths, exercise, knit, or just sit or lie in a new location, hoping to fall asleep there. Sometimes they lie on the floor and find that this helps. A third do nothing at all except lie in bed tossing and turning. Insomnia victims often call friends in order to overcome feelings of estrangement and distress. They might take medication, or turn to alcohol to help a return to slumber. Sometimes sex at the beginning of the night, or during the night, is used to try to bring on sleep. And, because nothing really seems to work, insomnia victims often become devoted fans of all-night talk shows. They hate to see the light of dawn because it marks the end of the possibility of sleep for that night.

Who Is the Insomniac?

Insomnia is no respecter of sex, social class, or nationality. Every kind of person has come to my office seeking help. On one recent morning a ninety-eight-year-old patient, aided by his nurse and leaning heavily on a cane, entered my office and sagged into the chair opposite me. His complaint, a chronic inability to sleep, was drug-induced, caused by misuse of sleeping medication. Later that afternoon, I was consulted by a mother who complained that neither she, nor her husband, could get any sleep because of their one-year-old child's inability to settle. In between, I saw a newly divorced woman in her forties, a machinist who suffered an injury on the job that he attributed to the aftereffects of a sleepless night, and a Wall Street broker who seemed ready to jump out of his skin.

I have been consulted by people from African states, by emigres from the Soviet Union, by individuals of Asiatic and Middle Eastern origin, as well as by citizens of many European nations.

The chronic insomniac, tossing restlessly in and out of light sleep or walking the floor to tire him- or herself out enough to be able to fall back to sleep, often feels alien and alone in the dark, surrounded, it seems, by an unseen sea of effortless sleepers. In fact, however, the prevalence of insomnia is astonishingly high. Surveys conducted in both the United States and Europe showed approximately one-third of the general population complaining of a current inability to sleep. Half of that number described the problem as so serious that they had sought professional help.

Chronic insomnia generally starts before the age of forty. It tends to begin earlier for those who have their major difficulty in falling asleep, while beginning a decade later for those with problems in staying asleep. Insomnia is also gender related, with a higher incidence among women. A study conducted in the European republic of San Marino showed twenty percent of people between forty and forty-four suffering from insomnia, with men and women affected about equally. However, between forty-five and fifty-four the prevalence in men rose only slightly, whereas that in women doubled. It is suggested that the large increase in the proportion for women results from difficulties arising from menopause.

Insomnia has also been found to be particularly prevalent in the following groups: those who are thin, older, anxious, or depressed; people who are suffering from medical illness or enduring recent life stress; and abusers of alcohol and other drugs.

The typical duration of chronic insomnia met in clinical practice is fourteen years, although I have encountered patients who had suffered for twenty-five years or more. This does not mean that insomnia is impervious to treatment; rather, it reflects the fact that treatments that work for many intractable cases have been developed only in the past decade. Most of the long-term sufferers I see have not previously been exposed to newer techniques and approaches; the great majority of them can, indeed, be helped on the basis of new developments in treatment.

Total Permanent Insomnia

Insomnia literally means not being able to sleep at all, but this is actually an extremely rare occurrence—so rare that only three or four totally sleepless individuals are known to the world at present. One case was described in a San Francisco newspaper in 1986. The man had not slept since World War II. Even with the help of drugs, all he could achieve was light drowsiness. Since he could not sleep, for many years he was able to hold down two full-time jobs simultaneously, working in a factory during the day and as a taxi driver at night. But his deteriorating condition gradually made it impossible to do more than light, occasional work and he had to give up both occupations.

Sleep Deprivation Research

Sleep scientists have conducted experiments with enforced sleep deprivation in order to understand the effects of losing sleep; eliminating either an entire night's sleep or selected phases of sleep, such as REM, to see what would happen. The world's record for tolerance to total sleep loss was eleven days and nights without sleep. Fatigue, instability, and then hallucinations and illusions occurred after a few days of total sleep loss, especially in more vulnerable older individuals or those prone to stress. In spite of these effects, most subjects still demonstrated an ability to do well on extremely complex and demanding tasks, including motor tests and certain kinds of problem solving. The finding, though, was relevant only for brief tasks or those for which subjects felt strong motivation. Lengthy, boring, and repetitive activities tended to suffer more from the effects of sleep loss.

Most people who suffer from sleep loss feel sleepy during the day and tend to nod off. Some are so aroused by their insomnia, however, that they complain they can't nap, no matter how tired they are.

Insomniacs show increased irritability during the day and describe themselves as washed out, tense, anxious, nervous, depressed, and unhappy. They are inattentive, socially withdrawn, accident prone, feel clumsy, easily intimidated, avoid others, and show mental slowness and lethargy. Physically they complain of tension headaches, gastrointestinal symptoms, and various pains and aches. Their symptoms are usually at their worst in the morning, in contrast to the normal sleeper who is fatigued and feels down only in the late afternoon. Sleep loss effects in insomniacs can plague their entire day.

Like the subjects of sleep deprivation experiments, typical insomniacs can often perform demanding work quite well for short periods of time, but they deal less well with repetitive assignments. Thus someone who must give a presentation at a professional or sales meeting may rise to the occasion, whereas another person performing repetitive and monotonous work encounters great difficulty.

As a rule, sleepiness after one night of poor sleep is not so severe that its effects in terms of fatigue, mood, and performance cannot be overcome. Even two consecutive nights of sleep deprivation need not cause trouble that can't be lived with. Two nights of poor sleep seems to be the cutoff point, however. After a third night, the symptoms become increasingly disturbing, and can be a sign of the beginning of a chronic pattern of sleep difficulties.

Causes of Insomnia

Insomnia is not an illness *per se*. Rather, it is a symptom with manifold causes, much like fever or headache.

There are numerous causes of insomnia. Dozens have been listed by sleep researchers and clinicians. When we separate this diverse list into several large categories—each based on related causes—it is possible to narrow down the probable roots. The major sources of insomnia are:

1. Stress, whether caused by a single traumatic event or continuing secondary effects of other conditions.

2. Medical problems, especially in the older population.

3. Psychological problems, often of a significant nature, that affect many areas of the patient's life.

4. Drugs, whether owing to misuse of prescription and over-the-counter preparations, or side effects from drugs prescribed for conditions other than insomnia, or from promiscuous street or recreational drug use.

5. Environment, including poor sleep hygiene (the topic of Chapter 8), persistent external disturbances, and sleep partner provocations.

6. Sleep disorders (such as those causing abnormal leg movements, or breathing difficulties during sleep, or narcolepsy) which are rooted in the malfunctioning of the nerve centers or neurochemical systems associated with sleep.

7. Faulty sleep associations, which occur in certain susceptible

individuals when confronted with an otherwise temporary period of sleeplessness. In such cases, a type of chronic sleep difficulty called "habit" or "conditioned" insomnia can be a grievous outcome.

8. Disturbances of circadian rhythms, the schedule of our wake–sleep action (and other biological functions), is another source of insomnia. The disruptions of sleep caused by jet lag, shift work, and irregular sleep patterns are examples.

Let's look more closely at these causes.

* * *

Stress is one of the most common causes of insomnia. Traumatic life experiences can be the trigger for insomnia at any age. Seventy-four percent of a group of poor sleepers reported that their first attack of insomnia coincided with a period of great stress. Social, interpersonal, emotional, economic, familial, or physical problems in our individual lives may be the source of stress. Most of us, unhappily, are acquainted with the experience of such distressing events as the loss of a loved one, the breakup of a love affair or marriage, the diagnosis of a major illness, the need for surgery, the calamity of a serious economic loss, or other traumatic misfortunes.

The loss of a job is a serious stressor. But, paradoxically, the responsibilities and pressures to succeed that come with a new position can also create acute insomnia.

Our response to stress is a state of arousal, and either we "fight or take flight." This response goes through the stages of alarm, resistance (the mobilization of resources), and exhaustion (if the stress demands on body, mind, or emotions are too much or last too long, we use up our reserves and, in a sense, break down).

The normal resiliency of most people enables them to deal with run-of-the-mill stress. When a person has the ability to adapt and has effective supporting networks, stress effects usually last only a short time. When insomnia is present, it is usually transient and short term. Such short term insomnias often flare up as the result of a single and quite obvious causal event and usually extinguish themselves after a few weeks of the inciting trauma.

When the stressor is very strong, or very lasting and serious in its implications, or when the coping ability of the individual is reduced, or when supporting networks are lacking or inadequate, the insomnia will tend to endure for a longer time, and evolve into a chronic condition. In predisposed individuals, even though the stressor diminishes or disappears, the sleep problem sometimes continues.

In other cases, the insomnia may eventually be overcome and disappear after a longer or shorter term. A recurrent or different stress down the road may cause the sleep problem, like an allergic reaction, to flare up again because a sensitivity has been created.

A prescription of tactics to reduce stress is presented in Chapter 9.

* * *

The entire gamut of medical problems, ranging from persistent but relatively secondary conditions (such as allergies, arthritis, or bladder problems) to grave cardiovascular or cancerous illnesses can cause insomnia. Pain or breathing difficulties are frequent sources of the problem. Stimulant drugs, or medical conditions, like hyperthyroidism and excessive adrenal activity, that cause hyperarousal can lead to sleeplessness. Hyperacidity, migraines, and other physiological reactions that are aberrantly activated during sleep, and that cause pain or other distress, are often important as origins of sleep problems.

Studies show that obesity, overeating, and anorexia have sleep effects. This is also true of some antibiotics and allergens. Another study shows that infants suffering from milk allergy sleep better when milk is eliminated from their diets.

* * *

People with psychological problems do not necessarily suffer from insomnia. Most people think they do, however, which is one reason why insomnia victims often take great pains to try to hide their sleep difficulties; they don't want to be labeled as being psychologically troubled. Sizable numbers of insomnias are caused by poor sleep hygiene (poor sleep practices), sleep disorders, aging, faulty conditioning, drugs, medical problems, and many other nonpsychiatric conditions. Nevertheless, the incidence of insomnia in psychiatric outpatients ranges from seventy-five percent during the acute phase of an episode, to one-third this amount during the followup period. Specialized sleep centers report psychiatric conditions (especially anxiety and depression) in thirty-five percent of patients who come to the clinics with a primary complaint of insomnia. In these cases, it is necessary to decide whether the insomnia is the result of a psychiatric problem and secondary to it, or whether the depression, anxiety, and other psychological symptoms are, in fact, an outgrowth of a longstanding insomnia. Insomnia itself may be a red flag, signaling the possibility of an underlying psychological or medical problem.

* * *

Drug withdrawal can create havoc with sleep patterns. This is true whether the withdrawal is from sleeping pills, self-administered over-the-counter drugs, or street and recreational drugs. This is primarily a problem of misuse.

Insomnia can also be a side effect which accompanies properly prescribed medications.

* * *

The impact of environmental influences on sleep, such as noise or temperature, can be a tantalizing question. It is easy to overcome an environmentally induced insomnia with a clearly discernable cause. It can sometimes be a real test of ingenuity to pinpoint exactly what it is in the environment that is creating the problem, however. It may be as simple as an early bird neighbor's front door slamming every weekday morning at four A.M. You were asleep and do not remember the slam; you only know that you are awakened and having trouble going back to sleep.

* * *

Organically based sleep disorders and conditioned insomnia are significant causal categories, and are discussed in detail in appropriate sections, as are the disturbances of circadian rhythms.

* * *

These categories of causes can, and often do, overlap in many cases of chronic insomnia, creating a knot of problems that must be disentangled in order to restore more normal sleep. This volume will deal with many of these complex situations. Despite the plethora of causes that exist for insomnia, my treatment approach significantly narrows down the search for the source of a sleep problem. The technique focuses on the identification of the particular type of sleep loss—whether it is difficulty in falling asleep, or staying asleep, or awakening too early. We will deal with the applications and value of this approach in the later chapters.

First, though, you should know something about the nature of "The Sleep World"—the realm of rest and recovery—that we enter every night of our lives; the topic of the next chapter.

Chapter 2

The Sleep World

What is this state of sleep? It has certain behavioral earmarks, such as relative immobility and quiet, as well as a heightened arousal threshold. It takes more stimulation to bring us out of sleep than to arouse us from relaxed wakefulness. At the same time, the state of sleep still permits rapid awakening to meet an emergency. Also associated with sleep are typical species-specific sleep positions in the lower orders, determined mainly by physiology. In human beings, however, our preferred sleep positions are determined by psychology and only secondarily by physiology.

Sleep is a different biological state than anesthesia, hibernation, or torpor. It is similar to other automatic, rhythmic body functions, like breathing, blood circulation, and digestion, that are relatively involuntary and regular.

Sleep is called "diurnal" if it occurs during the day, "nocturnal" if occurring at night, and "crepuscular" if occurring at dawn or dusk. If it has no particular pattern it is designated as "arrhythmic."

Sleep as humans know it began about 100 million years ago, when Australia, New Zealand, and the South Pacific Islands broke off from the main land mass. The mammals then existing "down under" continued an independent line of evolution thereafter in Australia and New Guinea, and their descendants now represent four or five distinct exotic species. Two varieties are spiny anteaters and the duck-billed platypus. These atypical mammals have unusual features. They are warm blooded like dogs, horses, and humans; yet, as do birds and reptiles, they bear their young through egg laying. Their sleep is also unique among mammals in that it is all of one type, what we now call nonrapid eye movement (NREM, pronounced "non-REM") sleep. All other mammals have two types of sleep, a phase of rapid eye movement (REM) sleep, as well as NREM sleep. Through extrapolation from this evolutionary marker the emergence of the distinctive type of human and mammalian sleep—identified by the two phases of NREM and REM sleep—was pinpointed in time.

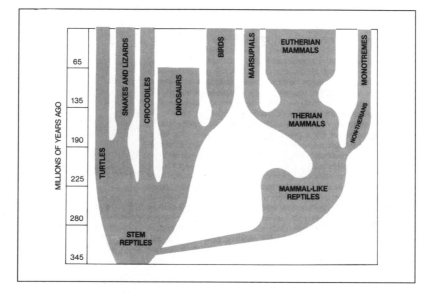

Evolutionary Lines of Living Reptiles, Birds and Mammals. Therians (most of the mammals) bear live children. Monotremes are egg-laying mammals whose few descendants (like the spiny anteater) are to be found (after the split off from the Asian land mass about 190 million years ago) in Australia and adjacent Southwest Pacific islands. These monotremes show non-rapid eye movement (NREM) sleep only. All other mammals have rapid eye movement (REM) and NREM sleep. (Reproduced with permission from Kryger M.H., T. Roth, W.C. Dement: *Principles and Practice of Sleep Medicine*, Philadelphia: W.B. Saunders, 1989, p. 33.)

Biological Clocks

Sleep is regulated by an internal biological clock. Our sleep–wake schedule, like dozens of other bodily processes, is a "biological rhythm" that functions in an on–off coordinated way. Our biological rhythms wax and wane, and are cued into the events of the typical day. We are awake and active during daylight and asleep during the dark of night.

Some of our biological clocks, like the one for sleep, operate on a twenty-four hour or full-day schedule, and are called circadian (*circa* means about, *dies* a day). Circadian rhythm is shown not only by our waking and sleeping but by our patterns of activity and idling, hormone production, body temperature, mood, mental performance, and many other physical and mental functions.

Ultradian rhythms have cycles that occur more often in the twenty-four hour period and are exemplified by NREM–REM rhythms, heart rates, meal times, and respiration and urination frequencies. Infradian cycles, such as the menstrual cycle, take place less often than circadian.

The study of our biological rhythms is now an important and valuable branch of physiology called "Chronobiology."

Our daytime activity is followed by a sleeping period, roughly on the basis of a formula of two-to-one—that is, sixteen hours of daytime activity followed by eight hours of nighttime sleep.

This rhythmic pulsing serves as an economic means of insuring the buildup of supplies and their availability without excessive wastage, as might occur if body functions were always in the "on position." Instead, supplies are available pretty much as needed, so that, for example, our temperature is high during the day when we most need our energy supply, and low at night when there is little demand.

This activity–rest cycle can proceed at different tempos, however. Under experimental conditions of isolation, such as in a mine, or in a laboratory room without any orientation to daylight or darkness, the true innate daily span of human activity and sleep emerges, and has been found to be approximately twenty-five hours, a one hour difference beyond actual clock time. Usually, without conscious knowledge, we adjust our body rhythm daily to eliminate that extra one hour, taking our time of day orientation from light or darkness, or from the numbers on a timepiece. The twenty-five hour span of our circadian rhythm, with its spare hour beyond the clock day, is seen as nature's way of giving us a little extra time in reserve to deal with seasonal changes in light and darkness and keep our internal clocks ticking smoothly.

The wake–sleep cycle of twenty-four hours is not firmly and irreversibly fixed. When isolation continues for an extended period and there are no time cues, people may even go on to operate on the basis of a thirty- or more hours-per-day cycle.

Our various body rhythms are turned on and off by centers that control their specific activities. One of the major achievements of sleep research has been the anatomical location of the master clock that regulates our circadian cycles. It was found to be a nucleus of cells that lies on the underside of the frontal part of the brain.

Some rhythms are quite flexible, being very amenable to changes of cue; waking and sleeping schedules are examples. The temperature rhythm, on the other hand, is fairly stubborn and not as easily shoved around. The pacing of cycles responds to cues from the environment. The cues we commonly use for setting wake–sleep and activity–rest times are light, temperature, mealtimes, and social activities. The technological advance of electric lighting, which enables our civilization to work night or day, has blurred the formerly dominant day and night pattern. This creates special problems for shift workers, submariners, and astronauts, as well as for those who live in regions like the subarctics that do not conform to our usual light–dark schedule.

Research on our patterns of sleepiness, mood, and performance has shown them to be biphasic, occurring at two times during the course of the day. Our major period for sleep and inactivity is at night, at least for people who lead a nine-to-five working existence. Approximately twelve hours ahead or behind the middle point of our sleep, however, people also show a decrease in vitality, tend to be moody, and are prone to a period of sluggishness. This usually occurs between two-thirty and four-thirty in the afternoon. For this reason folk wisdom has instituted the tradition of teatime or a coffee break for a pickup. In contrast to common belief, high noon and the time immediately following is not a period of drowsiness and siesta susceptibility. Rather, it is in the late morning and early afternoon when we are at our best and most alert. It is only at 7:30 to 9 P.M., in the normal day's schedule, that we get our second wind and recover our efficiency again after the afternoon dip. To ride with the wind, so to speak, we should schedule our activities and opportunities in harmony with these rhythmic patterns.

Unraveling Sleep's Mysteries: Modern Sleep Research

Good sleepers take these rhythms and sleep itself pretty much for granted. At the same time, however, human beings have always been intrigued by the mysteries of sleep, particularly dreams, and all the arts have made use of the associations between sleep and sex, as well as sleep and death. In Greek mythology the sleep god was called Hypnos. His twin, Thanatos, was the god of death, and Morpheus was the god of dreaming. The Roman god of sleep, Somnus, was seen as an ambiguous and somewhat sinister figure. In literature, from the ancient tale of Sleeping Beauty to Shakespeare's *Romeo and Juliet*, the mingled connections of sleep, sex, and death have been endlessly explored.

But it was not until well into the twentieth century, however, that the true scientific investigation of sleep began. Modern sleep research began with two major discoveries. In 1929, it was shown that electrical activity occurs in the brain and that it could be recorded, graphically charted, and studied. The development of the electroencephalographic (EEG) study of brain waves followed and, in the mid-1930s, led to the description of brain wave patterns associated with sleep.

The second major discovery took place in 1953, when the singular state of sleep associated with rapid eye movements, REM sleep, was revealed. It was found that the eyes moved periodically during sleep and that these REM periods were associated with a number of special events, such as dreaming, penile erections, and muscular paralysis. Since that time, the study of sleep has led to an explosion of important and exciting research, discoveries, and data.

It was found, with the description of dreaming REM sleep, and upon further investigation, that sleep occurred during the night in regular lawful cycles of four types of NREM sleep: stages 1 (marked by drowsy sleep), 2 (showing light sleep), and 3 and 4 (deep sleep). This NREM sequence was then followed by a period of REM (rapid eye movement) sleep. Such a complete NREM–REM cycle takes approximately ninety minutes. A typical night of sleep for an adult comprises four to five such regularly repeated cycles.

Sleep laboratory research extended our understanding of these sleep cycles and their associated phenomena. In a typical sleep laboratory, the individual's sleep is studied in a quiet, relaxed environment for one or more nights. During this period, brain waves and other sleep events and processes are charted continuously. For an average eight hours of sleep spent in the laboratory a recording is made that stretches for approximately one-quarter of a mile. This procedure is known as polysomnography. The brain waves are recorded by about two dozen dime-sized electrodes attached to the

skull by suction cups and, similarly, electrodes are placed at the
outer edges of each eye to record eye movements. Body muscular
activity is recorded by electrodes attached to chin muscles. Further
types of recordings are used to measure breathing, blood pressure,
temperature, cardiac action, movements of the chest and abdomen,
penile erections, and vaginal blood flow. Other specialized techniques of recording physiological and behavioral data are used, as
necessary, for the particular clinical or research information required.

NREM and REM Sleep

Movements during a normal night of sleep, including twelve full
body turns, usually occur before or immediately after REM periods
and take place about thirty to forty times a night. Body movements

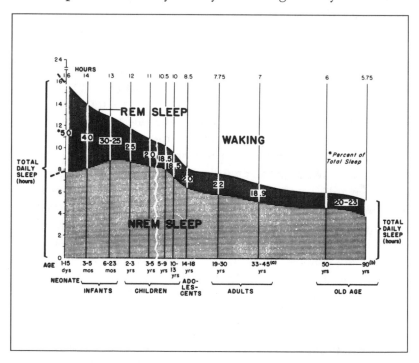

*REM (rapid eye movement) Sleep/NREM (non-rapid eye movement)
Sleep Relationship Throughout Human Life.* Shows the diminution of
REM sleep from 50 percent at birth to 20 percent in old age. NREM
remains more constant. Not shown is the loss of most deep NREM
(stages 3 and 4) that decrease as we grow older. (Reproduced with permission from Williams, R.L., I. Karacan, C.A. Moore. *Sleep Disorders:
Diagnosis and Treatment,* N.Y.: Wiley, 1988, p. 297.)

occur in the lighter stages of sleep, but not in deep 3 and 4 NREM and during REM paralysis.

As NREM progresses from stage 1 to stages 2, 3, and 4, perceptual sensitivity to the world diminishes progressively. It takes a very loud sound to arouse a sleeper in the last two stages, in contrast to, for example, stage 1, where merely a whisper may be sufficient. Vision fades with the onset of sleep, and we are functionally blind in both NREM and REM. It takes the largest amount of stimulation to wake an individual from stage 4 NREM. If we are awakened from the lighter stages of sleep we come awake fairly quickly, but it takes quite a while to awaken from deep NREM.

REM sleep is specifically characterized by coordinated eye movements and absolute paralysis of most voluntary muscles of the body except for faint flickerings of the lips and tips of the fingers and toes. Pulse, blood pressure, and brain cell activity, which have been throttled during NREM, increase sharply to levels equaling that of waking life. Blood, which had been pooled in the muscles during NREM, is now shifted to the brain. REM sleep has been characterized as a wakened brain in a paralyzed body. In NREM, the body is relaxed but not paralyzed and the brain is more or less asleep.

Sleep is usually initiated by a NREM cycle that contains the greatest amount of stage 3 and 4 sleep of the night. As stage 3 and 4 sleep is particularly refreshing, the old aphorism that sleep before midnight is the best has a physical basis. Taken together, these last two stages of NREM sleep are known as "delta" or "slow wave sleep." Their brain wave recordings (delta waves) are like rolling ocean swells, slow in speed and large in amplitude. Delta, or slow wave sleep is the deepest, most restorative part of all NREM. It is needed for replenishment, repair, and growth. For example, it is during this period that growth hormone is secreted. If slow wave sleep is excessively disturbed and hormone production seriously diminished during the growth period of childhood, dwarfism can result. During NREM, immunity medicators needed to fight infection, such as interferon, are released, which is why we feel better after a good night's sleep when we are ill.

REM sleep is thought to be intimately involved in memory and learning as well as the maintenance of emotion and mood.

As the night progresses, slow wave sleep diminishes, and the duration of REM sleep periods increases, going from about five minutes for the first REM period to about an hour for the last.

REM sleep constitutes about twenty-five percent of a typical night's sleep, most REM occurring in the last part of our sleep. The distinctive dreaming of REM sleep is accompanied by scanning movements of the eyes that sometimes seem to "follow" the activity in the dream.

Dreams also take place during NREM sleep but much less frequently, and are of a different nature: They are terser, less bizarre, more concrete, more everyday, and more tied to actual events.

Chapter 3

The Three Kinds of Insomnia

Discovering Your Type

Here is what would take place if you had insomnia and consulted me.

Your treatment would start with a comprehensive and intensive evaluation. This is crucially necessary in order to pinpoint the nature and possible origins of the sleep problem and to determine the appropriate treatment. It takes an hour, and usually more, to properly evaluate a case of chronic insomnia. Busy general physicians simply do not have the time for this procedure. In addition, the spectrum of skills required to evaluate and treat sleep problems are usually not within their range of expertise.

Until recently, when consulted about insomnia, doctors prescribed a sleeping pill, hoping to eliminate the complaint quickly, and at the same time warning against overuse of the medication. Today's well informed medical practitioners approach the problem differently to avoid unnecessary reliance on drugs. The accepted present practice is to review the possible causes of the sleep difficulty, and to suggest a practical way to deal with its assumed origin. In some cases, this advice may be coupled with a controlled short course of sleep medication. If these early steps are not effective, referral to a sleep specialist is the general procedure.

If I were the sleep clinician you consulted, I would see you for about an hour and a half for the initial workup. This procedure would include a detailed evaluation of the problem, a review of sleep hygiene guidelines, and instruction in the completion of sleep logs. Thereafter, I would see you approximately every two weeks for about five to six sessions.

The following questions are representative of the type of inquiries I make in my comprehensive workup in order to reach a diagnosis, causal formulation, and an appropriate treatment program.

You would be asked about how the insomnia began. Did it come out of the blue or gradually? How long has it lasted? Has it gotten worse or better? Are there any stressors that may have played a precipitating role in the current or previous episodes? The development of the problem would be traced.

I would be concerned whether the difficulty is falling asleep, staying asleep through the night, or awakening too early in the morning: the three basic kinds of insomnia.

Since insomnia is a daytime as well as a nighttime illness, I would check for daytime fatigue, sleepiness, poor concentration, performance falloff, and whether such ancillary effects of chronic insomnia as irritability, moodiness and depression, headaches, or muscle aches are present. You would be asked about nighttime awakenings, and whether they present any difficulties. I would ask you about clockwatching, and whether there are sleep worries during the day or in the presleep period.

The following step-by-step vignette will illustrate how your workup would proceed.

Hector Gonzalez, twenty-four years old and single, had been having sleep problems for the last six years, starting in college. He awakened frequently during the night and many times could not return to sleep. He often awakened an hour or two before the alarm. The problem got worse when he started working, about a year before coming to treatment. He was especially fatigued in the morning and sleepy throughout the day. His concentration was either wholly intact or, at times, almost absent. He watched the clock when he awoke at night. His fretful insomnia worries were present mainly during extended periods of sleep difficulty, increasing as bedtime approached.

I went back into archeological sleep time and asked about childhood and adolescent sleep patterns, looking for a history of early childhood sleep problems, like sleepwalking or sleep terrors. I also tried to find out if he was a "lark" or an "owl" at that early time.

Sleeping pill use, if any, was carefully reviewed, including the amount, frequency, side effects, and other pertinent information. I asked about any sleep aids that were used, in addition to sleeping pills, like sleep tapes, relaxation procedures, special dietary or homeopathic regimens, or any other mechanical or chemical aids or routines.

Hector's asthma, as a child, interfered with his sleep when he had attacks at night. The asthma disappeared after a few years but returned when he was in his early twenties.

He preferred to go to bed at a late hour all his life, and his mother described him as "time backwards." Otherwise, he had no other difficulties until junior high school, when his owl sleep pattern made it difficult for him to get up on school days. When asked about sleeping pills, he answered in the negative.

I noted his normal sleep parameters: the time of going to bed; "lights-out" time (LOT); "wake time" in the morning (WT); and the "total sleep time" (TST) that he felt was necessary for him to get a good night of sleep.

He was asked whether he experienced disturbed nighttime breathing, snored loudly, or had abnormal leg and body movements during sleep, excessive daytime sleepiness, sleep paralysis, or similar defining symptoms that would point to the possible existence of a major sleep disorder.

Hector's lights-out time was 1:30 A.M. His wake time was supposed to be 7:45 A.M. However, he often slept until 8:45 A.M. to catch up on sleep after a poor night and had to frantically rush to get to work, often getting there late. He was threatened with being fired for his chronic lateness. It was this threat that led him to consult me. Weekends he went to bed at 5:00 A.M. and slept till 1:00 P.M. His average sleep time during the week was six hours, giving him a daily sleep debt of two hours.

He did not give any evidence of suffering from a major sleep disorder, but reported that he had "nightmares" about fifteen to twenty minutes after the beginning of sleep and in the morning.

This part of the inquiry was followed by a review of his medical history; including a specific check for thyroid, adrenal, cardiac, arthritic problems, or any signs of other physical disorders that might have significance for sleep. I reviewed the type and amount of drugs that he might be taking for a medical condition, to evaluate the possible effects of such drugs on sleep.

Hector had had migraines since seventeen but had used no drugs for them. His asthmatic attacks were treated with an inhaler containing a stimulating antiasthmatic. He used an antihistamine occasionally, when his allergies for cats and grass flared up. He was not allergic to drugs.

Psychiatric status was reviewed and assessed; I reviewed the use of any psychotropic drugs. I weigh the relation of a psychiatric state—if one exists—to the outbreak of the insomnia, where this seemed relevant.

I checked his preferred sleep positions, both individual and couple (if the bed is shared with a partner). If the bed or bedroom is shared, I ask questions about partner-related influences, such as: Is your partner restless or an imperialist about bedcovers? Are there any partner-related practices that interfere with your sleep? Are you comfortable sharing the bed or bedroom? I inquire about preferences in the timing of sex, such as: Does your restlessness awaken your partner who then reacts by awakening you in turn? Does your partner snore, sleepwalk, sleeptalk, grind teeth, or otherwise wake you up? Do the two of you have sleep schedule incompatibilities, such as lark/owl or differing shift work schedules? If possible, it is always valuable to interview the sleep partner. This testimony is important in cases where the problem concerns hypersomnia, narcolepsy, sleep apnea, or depression, or when there is abuse of sleep medicine or other drugs. Partners are also important in maintaining compliance with a medication program and in serving as morning wakers, when necessary.

Hector shared a queen bed with his live-in girlfriend. His studio apartment was comfortable. Luckily, his girlfriend was also an owl and there were no partner-related sleep conflicts. Hector's preferred sleep position, which I successfully predicted from his history, was the Full-fetal.

Sleep Logs

Beginning with the first visit, you would be instructed on how to fill out sleep logs. The logs are organized on a weekly basis. They are reviewed in the biweekly visits, and serve as a graphic sleep diary. Insomnia has dozens of causes, and one of the primary purposes of using sleep logs is to help narrow down the search for the presumptive origin of the sleep difficulty.

The sleep log samples illustrated demonstrate the way logging helps classify the sleep loss pattern at issue. At the same time it highlights the possible origins of the sleep problem and points the way to effective treatment. Sleep logs should be completed within a half hour after waking, while the memory of the night's sleep is still fresh. It's important not to be rigid in completing the log, since

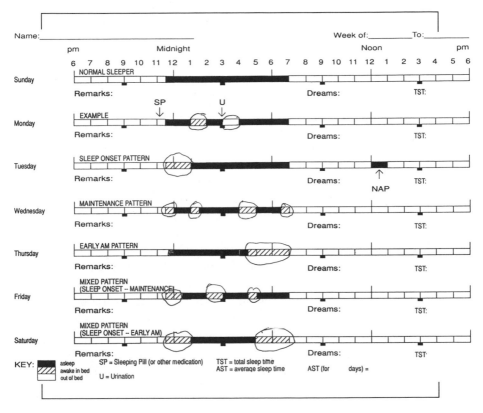

Samples of Completed Sleep Logs for Different Types of Insomnia.
Sunday shows normal sleep. Monday shows two patterns of middle sleep awakenings. In the first pattern, the person cannot sleep from 1 to 2 A.M. but remains in bed. In the second pattern, the person cannot sleep from 3 to 4 A.M. but gets out of bed. Tuesday shows charting of a sleep onset insomnia lasting 1½ hours from 11:30 P.M. to 1:00 A.M. Wednesday shows a sleep maintenance insomnia with prolonged awakenings during the night and some difficulty in both falling asleep and in awakening too early. Thursday shows a pattern of early A.M. insomnia, awakening 2½ hours too early. Friday shows a common mixed pattern of sleep onset and sleep maintenance insomnias. Saturday shows another mixed pattern, of sleep onset and early A.M. insomnias. Charting uses directions of the key at lower left. N.B. that naps are also charted and included in total sleep time.

the pattern is more important than the precision of the data. Sufficient details are usually available after at least two weeks of entries to be able to reach fairly reliable conclusions about the nature of the insomnia at hand.

Each line of the log shows a twenty-four hour day, from 6 P.M. of one day to 6 P.M. of the next, with the sleep period centered. Naps should be recorded in addition to the night's sleep. The key shows the three types of entry: The shaded portion is used for sleep, the diagonal portion for being in bed awake, and the blank portion for being out of bed. Total sleep time (TST) for each day is recorded to the right. Periods of less than a half hour can't be recorded within the limits of this form.

Average sleep time (AST), at the bottom, is the total hours of sleep for the period recorded, divided by the number of days. Remarks to the left of each day's line are used to briefly note relevant stresses or crises that might have influenced that night's sleep. Such crises might be: failing an examination; losing out on a business deal; quarreling with a spouse, parent, child, or friend; or worrying about an important matter scheduled to come up the following day. Dreams are to be recorded to the right if space allows; if not, they can be completed on the opposite side of the form. Sleeping pills, or other medication that might have an impact on your sleep, are shown at SP (for sleeping pills) with an arrow to indicate the time taken. The notation of the pills taken should include the dosage amount. Urination during the night is shown by the letter U at the time of occurrence. An important point is to be sure to include naps in the logging regardless of when they occur, since naps are included in reckoning your total daily sleep amount.

The Three Kinds of Insomnia

Sleep loss may occur as either a Sleep Onset Insomnia, with difficulty in falling asleep at the beginning of the night; as a Middle (or Maintenance) Insomnia, with midsleep awakening or awakenings, often characterized by great difficulty in falling back to sleep, and sometimes lasting through the remainder of the night; or as Early A.M. (for early morning) Insomnia, with premature morning awakening at one to four hours before normal wake time.

The completed sleep log illustrates different patterns of insomnia. Tuesday demonstrates a sleep onset insomnia, Wednesday shows middle insomnia, and Thursday shows early A.M. insomnia. Two mixed types of insomnia are also shown; the quite common sleep onset and middle insomnia combination, and the combination of a sleep onset and an early A.M. insomnia.

With the latter type—early A.M. insomnia—it is important to be aware that it can sometimes occur as early as in the middle of the sleep period and last through the rest of the night, although it usually begins an hour or two before wake time.

Hector's sleep log analysis showed a sleep onset insomnia pattern with a long sleep onset latency of from forty minutes to an hour. He had a tendency for late bedtimes; he often went to bed at 2:30 A.M. or later. Yet, despite this delayed lights-out time it still took him almost an hour to fall asleep. Since he had to awaken when the alarm went off, he could only sleep about four hours, dangerously indulging in catchup sleep and being late to work. He would try to make up his sleep debt by sleeping nine or more hours on weekends.

The graphic picture that logs give of the type of sleep loss that is present can be very enlightening if you are one of the sleep deprived. In addition to the knowledge and valuable insights gained from this record keeping, a feeling of helpless victimization can be relieved by the very act of charting. The ability to see the patterns that exist in your sleep problem helps to dilute the feelings of passivity and helplessness that are a corollary of chronic insomnia. Charting can also show you how frequently a correlation exists between a given crisis you might be undergoing and the sleep difficulties you are likely to experience that night.

In addition to providing a quantitative estimate of the amount of sleep loss, the logs also serve as a baseline for the improvement, or lack of improvement, that follows a given treatment.

Of course, these logs should be kept during normal everyday periods, and should not be used during vacations or business trips. These events introduce too many atypical and complicating factors for reliable use of the sleep log.

The log can also heighten your awareness of the need to adhere to a fixed schedule of lights-out and wake times.

Using the log, I calculate the average total sleep time for each night. It is amazing how consistent these average total sleep times are when charted in this way!

In Hector's case he averaged only a six and one-quarter hour total for a night's sleep. This sleep loss of about two hours daily accounted for his chronic tardiness, sleepiness, and fatigue.

Treatment Recommendations

Treatment recommendations for insomnia can be general, as when good sleep hygiene guidelines are outlined, but it usually has to be more specific. Ideally, the preferred way to free you from the problem is to determine the specific cause of your sleep loss and eliminate it. Insomnia treatment is usually a custom made product, identifying the particular pattern of insomnia, its roots, and determining the specific ways to overcome it.

My treatment method starts with this identification of the particular type of sleep loss—whether initial, middle, or early A.M. insomnia. This typing significantly narrows down the search for probable etiology, and the necessary treatment plan.

To illustrate, if we are dealing with an initial sleep onset insomnia I assume that the probable cause is one of the following: the effect of a conditioning process that results in sleeplessness; a high arousal level caused by an ongoing life stress; an anxiety generating conflict; an exaggeration of obsessional thinking; the effects of a heightened biological arousal caused by a high thyroid or adrenal level; medications, like steroids, that have stimulant properties; or a manifestation of a normally hyperaroused "Type A" personality. A limited number of other options are also considered; for example, a delayed or irregular sleep schedule (as in Hector's case), poor sleep hygiene, disruptive environmental influences, the presence of an atypical type of depression—Seasonal Affective Disorder or depression occurring in a young adult.

If you suffer from a middle insomnia picture, I consider the following probable sources: a drug-induced effect involving misuse of sleeping medication; medical problems, like asthma or ulcers that flare up during sleep; certain sleep disorders, like restless legs, or the apneas, or REM Dream Disorder, that are associated with middle insomnia; age with its lightened sleep; or the effects of alcohol.

With an early A.M. insomnia the probable causation is more circumscribed—a depression in some form. The possible existence of a circadian rhythm disturbance or of environmental sleep disruptive events must also be considered.

In order for you to identify your own insomnia pattern and its significance, I suggest that you fill out the two weeks of blank sleep logs, discover your own type, and make some speculations about its cause. The logs are to be filled in daily, within fifteen minutes after waking. Completion should use diagrammatic key at lower left of log: Black for sleep; diagonals for periods of lying in bed awake; and blank for being out of bed. Total sleep (TST) for a week is calculated by summing up all black spaces. Average sleep time (AST) is calculated by dividing the TST by the number of days charted.

To illustrate how this identification will help to pinpoint a probable cause of your insomnia, as it did successfully in Hector's case, let us turn to in depth discussions of the nature and treatment of the three kinds of insomnia and some of their common variants.

Name: _____

Week of: _____ To: _____

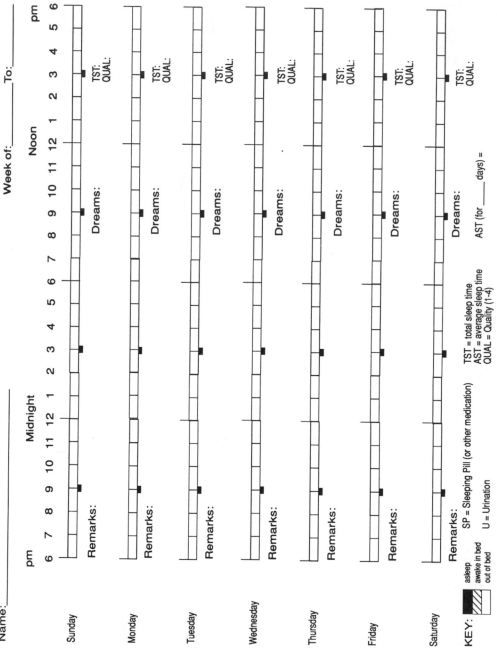

	pm					Midnight											Noon						pm
	6	7	8	9	10	11	12	1	2	3	4	5	6	7	8	9	10	11	12	1	2	3	4	5	6

Sunday
Remarks: Dreams: TST: QUAL:

Monday
Remarks: Dreams: TST: QUAL:

Tuesday
Remarks: Dreams: TST: QUAL:

Wednesday
Remarks: Dreams: TST: QUAL:

Thursday
Remarks: Dreams: TST: QUAL:

Friday
Remarks: Dreams: TST: QUAL:

Saturday
Remarks: Dreams: TST: QUAL:

KEY:
asleep
awake in bed
out of bed

SP = Sleeping Pill (or other medication)
U = Urination

TST = total sleep time
AST = average sleep time
QUAL = Quality (1-4)

AST (for _____ days) =

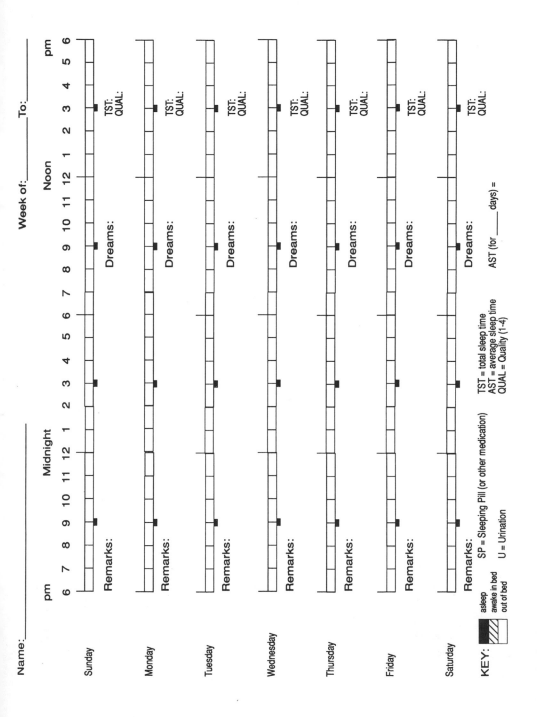

Name: _____

Week of: _____ To: _____

pm | **Midnight** | **Noon** | **pm**

6 7 8 9 10 11 12 1 2 3 4 5 6 7 8 9 10 11 12 1 2 3 4 5 6

Sunday
Remarks: Dreams: TST:
    QUAL:

Monday
Remarks: Dreams: TST:
    QUAL:

Tuesday
Remarks: Dreams: TST:
    QUAL:

Wednesday
Remarks: Dreams: TST:
    QUAL:

Thursday
Remarks: Dreams: TST:
    QUAL:

Friday
Remarks: Dreams: TST:
    QUAL:

Saturday
Remarks: Dreams: TST:
    QUAL:

AST (for ____ days) =

KEY:

■ asleep
▨ awake in bed
□ out of bed

SP = Sleeping Pill (or other medication)
U = Urination

TST = total sleep time
AST = average sleep time
QUAL = Quality (1-4)

Chapter 4

Sleep Onset Insomnia

A common form of chronic insomnia is difficulty in falling asleep. If this interval takes more than thirty minutes, Sleep Onset Insomnia—also called Initial Insomnia—is present. Sleep clinicians use the technical term "Sleep Onset Latency" to describe the length of time it takes to fall asleep. It is important to differentiate it from mere presleep lying in bed. How can we actually mark the beginning of an attempt to sleep? This is a subjective judgment of the point at which we first make up our minds to enter the sleep world. Even when the demonstration of will is rather minimal, as in allowing the book you are reading to slip from your hands while nodding off, the determination of sleep onset latency begins with the time of the decision to surrender to sleep. This is known as "lights-out time," the juncture at which, like the surfer looking for the right wave, you are poised awaiting the arrival of sleep.

The average sleep onset latency ranges from eight to fifteen minutes in good adult sleepers. In this interval most people are in the alpha state, resting with their eyes closed. Sleep onset latency is quite constant across the age spectrum, being the same from three to seventy, and rising only slightly in the years above seventy.

Both good sleepers and insomniacs tend to overestimate the length of time it takes them to fall asleep. Chronic poor sleepers suffering from sleep onset insomnia have been found to take three times as long to fall asleep as good sleepers. Since their temperature rhythm is also delayed for a similar period, this results in an inability to fall asleep during this interval. We are only able to descend into sleep when our temperature gradient begins to drop. For this reason, the hours immediately before the beginning of the nightly temperature fall is known as the "Forbidden Zone"—when sleep is out of the question.

The amount of sleep latency onset time for each individual seems to be fairly consistent and, although varying from night to night, shows a stable amount of initial sleep loss when calculated on a weekly basis. The average age at which a sleep onset problem begins is thirty-two years, somewhat earlier than in the other types of chronic insomnia.

Types of Sleep Onset Insomnia

Cases of sleep onset insomnia fall into a discrete number of categories that can be separated from one another by their cause, history, or by certain differentiating characteristics.

There are many insomniacs who strive for perfection and control in everything they do. Even in their quest for sleep they cannot "take their mind off their mind." When confronted with problematic or stress situations, they cannot leave worrying behind when the bed beckons. Their minds struggle with the need to overcome their daytime difficulties and their thinking will not let go even at lights-out time. This mental struggle results in an arousal that leads directly to loss of sleep capacity. In my experience, these personalities prefer to fall asleep in the prone position, lying on their stomachs. The picture of their lives shows preoccupation with orderliness, rigidity, rules, determination, and organized activity. Any perceived or threatened loss of orderliness or control becomes a worrying event that can extend into the night hours, preventing sleep. Good sleep hygiene (beneficial habits that promote sleep, the subject of chapter 8), especially establishing adequate wind-down time, and the use of effective stress reduction and relaxation tactics (see chapter 9) is the proper course in dealing with this situation.

A second personality with a tendency to have sleep onset problems I call the "High Arousal Type." These people seem to have a higher energy level than most of us. They are constantly in overdrive, both mentally and physically. Their driving nature will not let go even at night. In the evening hours, rather than relaxing and preparing for sleep, they occupy themselves with personal and business phone calls, do office work, balance the home books, and are socially overactive. As a result, they just can't stop to unwind as bedtime approaches. This temperament has been defined in the psychiatric literature as a "Type A Personality." Although many of them are good sleepers, a significant number find it difficult to turn off the on switch and shut down when entering the bedroom. Some of these hyperarousal types have high blood levels of activating hormones that are the result of glandular oversecretion, as in hyperthyroidism. Using prescribed stimulating drugs, such as steroids, causes hyperarousal in others.

Stress reduction, good relaxation practices, and sleep hygiene awareness are helpful here as in the previous example of the worrisome sleep losers. Consultation with their medical practitioners about biological or drug arousal problems may lead to the solution of their sleep disruption.

Another substantial group of sleep onset sufferers who experience problems falling asleep have chronic high levels of anxiety. Their history shows a tendency for anxiety episodes during the day, with attacks of rapid heartbeat, fear, agitation, sweating, dizziness, shortness of breath, and other physiologic manifestations of this emotional state. The anxiety may be moderate in degree or as intense as a panic attack. Whether constant (as in generalized anxiety), or occasional (as in a phobic episode or a stress period associated with fear), it interferes with sleep.

There are two special anxiety syndromes that are noted for their sleep disturbances. In Panic Disorder, patients experience severe anxiety attacks during sleep as well as during the day. The night attacks occur in NREM rather than in REM sleep, as with typical nightmares, and give rise to problems in falling asleep, awakenings, and fragmented sleep.

Posttraumatic Stress Disorder Syndrome occurs after a catastrophe, such as an earthquake, a crime experience, or a similar atypical traumatic event. Victims experience frightening flashbacks of the trauma, and live in a high state of constant arousal. This sets the stage for difficulties in sleep onset. In addition, they experience flashbacks during the night in the form of frightening anxiety dreams that repeat the trauma.

Good sleep hygiene discipline and stress reduction and relaxation tactics are helpful in the presence of an anxiety problem. If further help is necessary, the use of community and professional mental health resources is advisable. There are excellent techniques and facilities currently available to overcome anxiety problems.

Other possible origins of sleep onset difficulties are: a delayed sleep phase syndrome (the night owl pattern, see chapter 11 about this problem); drug actions, especially stimulants; and sleeping pill abuse that is linked to the development of tolerance (discussed in chapter 10).

Tinnitus, an annoying buzzing in the ears, is generally masked during wake time by the sounds of surrounding daytime activities. In the stillness of the bedroom, the ringing, piping, and wheezing of a case of tinnitus is heard, interfering with the ability to fall asleep—whether at bedtime or after midsleep awakenings.

Like tinnitus, hypnic jerks sometimes cause difficulty when people are trying to fall asleep. Normally a hypnic jerk (a sudden twitch of the entire body) can happen when we are falling asleep but is of low intensity and unperceived. In some persons the twitching is so frequent it prevents sleep. A high arousal state sets the stage for this phenomenon. Relaxation training, tranquilizers, or exploration of the sources of anxiety behind its appearance are methods of dealing with this problem.

The advent of the computer age has brought with it another source of sleep onset difficuties. Computer hackers, enjoying the play of technology during night hours, may become so aroused that falling asleep easily is impossible. Hackers should be aware of the effects of this disregard of good sleep hygiene and should correct the practice.

Conditioned or Psychophysiologic Insomnia

Another form of sleep onset insomnia, one of the most common, is associated with difficulty in falling asleep. It is called "Conditioned" or "Habit" Insomnia, or in sleep diagnostic classification, "Persistent Psychophysiologic Insomnia." A conditioning process is assumed to be the etiology. In Pavlov's classical experiment in learning, a bell was rung when a dog was presented with food. At the sight of food the dog began salivating. He soon learned that the ringing was associated with food. Later, Pavlov was able to elicit salivation in his experimental dog merely by the ringing of the bell without the actual presentation of food. In other words, the dog associated the ringing with food and responded as though the food would soon be there.

Similarly, in conditioned insomnia, after a period of poor sleep caused by some stress, predisposed individuals will thereafter associate poor sleep with the experience of their bedroom. Whenever confronting their beds they respond, like Pavlov's dog, with the expectation that they will be unable to relax and sleep. This association arouses them so much that, in fact, they become aroused and unable to sleep.

People who tend to experience this conditioned sleeplessness have a tendency to handle stress with internalization; repressing the feelings and conflicts linked to their stress-inducing situations. Instead of worrying about the actual conflicts embodied in the stress, they focus entirely upon the struggle for sleep. By doing this they create a sleep neurosis tied to a state of conditioned arousal. When they come to the office complaining about their dilemma, they enumerate intense efforts at achieving sleep. Their concentration on winning the battle with the sandman is all-consuming. As a result, they are unable to step back and look at the original stress that eventually resulted in the sleep problem.

Some inherently poor sleepers experience a night or two every month when they have difficulties. If they are exposed to an extended period of sleep loss caused by some stress, they may, as perfectionistic or anxious individuals, overreact to a "normal" episode of poor sleep that follows with the fearful expectation that it portends an extended period of insomnia. In this way, they create a reactive stress for themselves that reinforces their tendency to sleeplessness and sets the stage for the onset of a prolonged sleep difficulty. Their gloomy self-fulfilling prophecies are now realized by a vicious cycle of expectation, arousal, and insomnia.

Here we see a topsy-turvy play of effects. Originally stress may have created a temporary insomnia. Insomnia creates an extended stress with the newly aroused anxious expectation of sleeplessness; a complete reversal.

Insomniacs suffering from this form of sleeplessness are kept in a state of continual tension at bedtime. During the day they function quite well. As a rule, there is no picture of a frank neurosis in their psychologic patterns. Their conditioned sleeplessness has an independent life of its own, and does not correlate strongly and directly with day-to-day conflicts. When they have psychological distress, they blame it on their intractable insomnia problem.

Although conditioned insomnia is a unique type, it has an almost parasitic tendency to graft itself onto other insomnias, like those caused by anxiety and depression. When this happens, insomnia becomes the entire focus of fearful concern. The preoccupation with sleeplessness becomes an astronomical black hole, swallowing up all the original emotional conflicts. Characteristically, the harder these sleep losers try to sleep, the more difficult it is to succeed.

A classic discriminating sign of psychophysiological insomnia is that these sleep victims sleep better away from their own bedrooms. This occurs because their conditioned associations are absent in the new venue.

A patient of mine who suffered from this form of insomnia would look forward joyfully to traveling to another city. During the day he would wander around in the strange new city as though in a rich, delightful fantasy world. He loved every sight and sound of the surroundings, knowing that that night, when he went to bed, he would be able to sleep like a proverbial baby.

Conditioned insomniacs not only sleep well outside their own bedrooms, but even in a different bedroom in the same house or on the floor, rather than in their own beds. They show a paradoxical "first night effect" when seen in sleep laboratory investigations. In contrast to other testees, they sleep well in the sci-fi-like setting, and are embarrassed that they fall asleep so easily in these unusual surroundings when they have so much difficulty doing so at home. They have a tendency to nod off at the movies, or watching television, or at a lecture, or anywhere that the negative stimulus of their own bedroom, and its own arousing expectation of not being able to sleep, is absent.

The treatment of this insomnia is multidirectional. Desensitizing them from the negative conditioning requires them to limit their experience of struggling with their associations to the bed.

This technique, called "Stimulus Control" (described in detail in the Appendix) achieves release from the sleep inhibiting conditioning.

A second way of dealing with conditioned insomnia is emphasizing positive sleep hygiene practices and combining this with relaxation techniques. These tactics may be sufficient to remove the bed and bedtime as sources of stress. Recourse to hypnotics, on occasion, when sleep loss is severe, can also help overcome the feeling of dread and arousal found in this form of insomnia.

Other special techniques, such as "Paradoxical Intention," (also described in the Appendix) have shown effectiveness in reducing a conditioned sleep difficulty.

In other cases of sleep onset insomnia, the emphasis is on dealing with the particular cause of the difficulty and eliminating it. In generalized anxiety states this can mean antianxiety medication during the day that will carry over into the evening hours and reduce anxiety that may be causing the sleep onset problem. When pain is present and prevents falling asleep, amelioration of the condition causing the pain, plus the use of analgesics, when indicated, can be effective.

Behavior techniques, like stimulus control, are comparatively easy to understand. Strong motivation and willpower are required, however, as a rule. This is necessary to overcome the initial chagrin of an insomniac who experiences an increase of sleeplessness during the first days these measures are taken—since they require the abandonment of hypnotics, naps, and catchup sleep. For this reason, as in the parallel example of dieters attempting to reduce their weight, it is helpful to have counselors act as supporting backup during this trying time.

Focused Psychotherapy–Counseling Treatment

As a rule, although behavior techniques are highly effective in treating many types of chronic insomnia, this approach does not deal with underlying conflicts or stresses that interfere with sleep, and are frequently present. By far the most effective and longest lasting results in dealing with insomnia-engendering mental conflicts are achieved by focal short term psychotherapy. In these instances, short term focused psychotherapy–counseling can eliminate insomnia, restore good sleep, and have other beneficial effects. This treatment modality is within the range of skills of a large number of trained therapists and counselors, who, although not fully knowledgeable about sleep medicine, can be available to effectively treat conflict-based insomnia.

Of course, when counselors are not informed about sleep medicine, it is best that the evaluation and management of the sleep problem be under the aegis of a sleep professional; to avoid overlooking the possible presence of a complicating sleep disorder.

In focused psychotherapy, the insomnia victim can learn to express anger and other emotions appropriately, and to deal with repressed feelings. This removes the need to displace a stressful conflict onto a pattern of insomnia.

The following two clinical vignettes from my own practice illustrate the use and benefits of short term focused psychotherapy–counseling in dealing with conflict insomnia.

Helene Foxe, an executive in her thirties, developed a sleep onset insomnia characterized by severe difficulty in falling asleep. The history suggested a linking of the development of her insomnia with difficulties in a work relationship with a male superior. She herself had made this correlation and had changed jobs, but even this did not eliminate her insomnia problem.

In the course of our third session she related the following dream. She reported finding herself in a basement. Looking out through the windows, she saw a menacing dog prowling around her cellar fortress. The dream terrified and awakened her.

In the following session she associated this dream with an older brother who was arrested for exhibitionism. The dog represented the display of his aggressive animality and her fear of it. In some ways the male superior with whom she was in conflict resembled her brother and, for many reasons, this association aroused her anxiety.

With the dream recital—and her associations to it—the patient's anxiety dramatically disappeared along with her insomnia. This case illustrates the importance of discovering and dealing with the precipitating conflicts that cause an insomnia. In this example, the origin of her difficulties became clear rather quickly. In other cases the search may take a somewhat longer time. This is illustrated in the following case report.

Harry Conacker, a married corporate executive, was in his early fifties when he consulted me. His difficulties began after a kidney stone attack. Somehow, the surgical procedure to retrieve the stone resulted in painful physical complications. Even after removal of the stone he was faced, unfortunately, with further episodes of stone formation. These were determined to be a manifestation of an underlying endocrine disorder. All the subsequent stones passed spontaneously after short, moderately painful episodes, but he was left in dread of the possibility of another surgical procedure that would be as intensely painful as the first.

The anticipation of a recurrence of severe pain began to haunt his sleep. He would awaken numerous times during the night, sweating and panicky. He would find it difficult to fall asleep again after these awakenings, and would frequently be up for the remainder of the night.

Relaxation training, sedating antidepressants, and intermittent hypnotics provided only minimal relief.

In time, the content of our sessions gradually assumed more of a focal psychotherapeutic–counseling nature as we began to search for psychologic correlations between his surgery and his anxiety at night. The history and our ongoing discussions revealed the following significant life determinants behind his problem.

He was the only child of a weak but loving mother and a cold, stern, rigid father who never praised him but was cruelly critical if he made an error, although he was never actually physically abused by his father. His parents divorced when he was four and, since his mother had to go to work, he went to live with his grandparents, who loved him and showered him with affection and healthy emotional nurturing. This paradise ended when his grandmother died four years later. His mother was still single and working and his father had remarried in the interim. The only recourse in these changed circumstances was to live with his father. His stepmother and father had two small children. Within this family, despite the limited and rationed warmth of the stepmother, he was forced to return to a fear-laden existence until he grew up and was able to leave his father's roof.

In his mature years he had a bad marriage, was divorced, and finally found happiness with his second wife. He was secure in his job as a midlevel manager in a large company and his life proceeded placidly. The traumatic episode of stone removal, followed by intractable sleep distress, became an earthquake that shattered this orderly life.

His dreams showed themes of being followed and threatened by large sinister figures. Our discussions increasingly focused on his problems with his father and his anger with him. The concentration on this core conflict eventually led to an insight that centered on his relations with his employees.

As part of his duties at work, he conducted educational seminars with his staff. He presented the material in a manner that was dry and formal, imparting information in a lecture format with no discussion. He was always somewhat chagrined to notice the lack of response to his didactic efforts.

It was during the course of his work with me that his company sent him to attend a training program in educational methods. Here, he experienced the give and take of a learning technique that used interactive group process to transmit information in a stimulating way.

When he returned to his company afterward, he decided to employ a similar technique to instruct his staff. He was gratified to see an electrifying response to his new approach, with excited participation by the formerly glum members of his group.

The recitation of this experience covered a few sessions. At this point he announced that he was now feeling better, and treatment was terminated. His anxiety level was down and sleep was much better. The treatment had lasted twenty-two sessions.

The six-month followup revealed that he had slept well every night in the interim, needed no sleeping pills, and was feeling happy again. What caused this beneficial turn of events? Obviously, in his prior relations with his assistants he had been identifying with his authoritarian father. It was the focused sessions with me that finally allowed him to bring this basically false self into question and left him open to the enlightenment of the training program that transformed him. Instead of a pedant, he became a warm and relating person to the employees. The insight he reached finally enabled him to confront his feelings about his father and free himself from the anxiety-laden associations that were reawakened by his passive, painful victimization during the surgery. It was this painful reminiscence that had caused his insomnia.

Chapter 5

Middle Insomnia

Middle Insomnia (or Maintenance Insomnia), is difficulty in remaining asleep once the sleep journey through the night has begun. This dilemma of awakening and being unable to recapture sleep may occur only one time, or repeat itself during the night.

If the wakefulness lasts less than seven minutes, it will usually be forgotten. The disruptive effects of a single long awakening, or those of several repeated periods of wakefulness, will be manifested in insomnia symptoms the following day.

Very often sleep is lost for periods of an hour or two. When sleep returns, it is caused by accumulated weariness. This relief may be cruelly followed by another prolonged wake after a short and unsatisfactory interim sleep. It is also quite common for the sleep interruption to last throughout the balance of the night. The weary traveler through the dark will then attempt to recover some restfulness by catchup sleep in the early hours of morning. This maneuver is dangerous. It can lead to oversleeping.

In middle insomnia, staying awake involuntarily in midsleep seems much more painful to insomniacs than difficulties in falling asleep at bedtime. This is understandable, since the struggle to fall asleep in middle insomnia frequently must be mastered many times, in contrast to the single attempt needed in other types. Since the ability to fall asleep again is never completely predictable for them, middle insomnia victims feel like perpetual losers in Las Vegas.

Most episodes of middle insomnia begin about an hour and a half to two hours after the beginning of sleep, following the first full sleep cycle. The reason may be that it is easier to awaken from

REM, which occurs at this time, than from the typically deep initial NREM period that precedes it. Perhaps this is owing to the partial arousal of REM sleep, with its high levels of active biological and mental processes.

What May Be at Fault if You Have Middle Insomnia?

Middle insomnia is most often drug induced, the result of misuse of sleep medication. With repeated use of drugs, the body develops a "tolerance," an immunity to the actions of a drug which, in a sleeping pill, prevents sleep promoting action. The body attempts to offset the chemically induced effects of the sleeping pill with tolerance, and to restore the physiological status quo. When using hypnotics, the onset of the tolerance reaction will cause an arousal, and consequent awakening, instead of sedation and sleep. After a while, the exhausted victim, who is relying on pills that won't work, may succeed in falling asleep; but a seesaw battle, with repeated episodes of sleep disturbance during the night can ensue. A debilitating routine often develops, with the insomnia sufferer increasing the nightly amount of sleep medication, and the trained body quickly responding with tolerance. In the end, the tolerance reaction is so quick and strong that insomnia sets in almost at once. The sleep that is regained thereafter is very fragile and easily disrupted again. (For discussion of drugs and sleep, sleeping pills, and drug withdrawal tactics see chapter 12.)

The second major cause of middle insomnia is the effect of age-related sleep changes. This predicament is covered in chapter 14, which deals with the sleep problems of older people. If you find that you are spending too much time in bed in an attempt to overcome the effects of losing sleep caused by long awakenings during the night, use the method of Sleep Restriction (described in detail in the Appendix) to overcome this problem.

Certain sleep disorders cause difficulties in sleep maintenance. Restless legs and jerky legs are abnormal feelings and movements in the lower limbs that disturb sleep and are frequent causes of middle insomnia. (These disorders are covered in chapter 12.)

Other sleep disorders give rise to midsleep insomnia. An example is Alpha-delta Sleep, a sleep disturbance diagnosed by polysomnography, that shows the abnormal, sleep fragmenting presence of EEG alpha rhythms (a sign of wakefulness) during deep

NREM sleep. It is frequently associated with fibrositis, a rheumatic disease whose symptoms are musculoskeletal pain and tender body points. It has also been found in rheumatoid arthritis and pain syndromes. Tricyclic antidepressants relieve the condition.

Hypnic jerks that occur after awakening at night, may prevent being able to fall back to sleep. Anxiety states may also produce this sad effect. Use stress reduction and relaxation methods and good sleep hygiene to help. See the previous chapter about dealing with anxiety.

Sleep terrors in both children and adults are partial arousals out of NREM—like sleepwalking and sleeptalking—that take place in the early part of the night. See chapter 13 for a full discussion of this topic.

Secondary enuresis is the term for adult bedwetting. Like other parasomnias that occur in adults, it is precipitated by psychologic conflict. Adult enuresis may, however, also be a complication of diabetes or a neurological problem. Psychotherapy, to treat its psychogenic origin, is the preferred treatment. Successful treatment removes the symptom.

Dream-interruption insomnia causes awakenings during REM. These occur periodically and precisely every sixty to ninety minutes, during REM phases. They result from a state of severe anxiety that penetrates REM. Dreams, usually anxiety laden, may or may not be recalled from these episodes. They can be curbed by sedating REM suppressing drugs and counseling.

Another sleep problem with a psychogenic conflict base is receiving increasing notice. It occurs in young adults, both male and female, as well as in some middle-aged individuals. In this condition, a psychologically induced spasm of the voice-box muscles results in choking, gasping, and irritation of the throat that awakens the patient. Treatment is psychotherapy to deal with the stress-causing real life conflict.

Medical conditions, such as arthritis, heartburn caused by hyperacidity and gastroesophageal reflux, cardiac pain, and asthmatic attacks, as well as breathing disturbances resulting from lung and cardiovascular problems, are major sources of middle insomnia. Neurological and endocrine disorders are also common precipitants. Proper medical consultation is the correct course for these problems. See your doctor.

It is important to keep in mind that when medications are prescribed for medical problems, they can have side effects that interfere with sleep.

In heavy smokers, the emergence of nicotine withdrawal symptoms after two and a half to three hours into sleep can be responsible for a middle insomnia. Similarly, alcohol drunk in the presleep period loses its sedative qualities later, causing withdrawal effects and consequent awakening a few hours after imbibing, especially in chronic drinkers. (See chapter 8 on Sleep Hygiene.)

Environmental events should be considered in middle insomnia. Very frequently the source of discomfort, such as a noise occurring during the night, may not be perceived in sleep but can cause awakening. In addition to noise, such environmental factors as unrestful beds, and sleep disturbing temperature or light, may interfere with a restful night and result in awakenings. Try to identify these possible sources of sleep disruption and correct appropriately.

Chapter 6

Early A.M. Insomnia

It was late twilight when the thirty-five-year-old woman entered the offices of Insomnia Medical Services in New York. The approaching shadows of evening accentuated the lines on her haggard face. When she sat, I could scarcely distinguish the features of her face because her head was bent so low. I had to strain to hear her weak answers to my questions as she struggled to concentrate on the interview while fighting off an overwhelming desire to sleep.

Nicole Butterfield graphically evinced many of the main features of insomnia: drowsiness with a marked tendency to fall asleep, obvious fatigue, poor concentration, passivity, withdrawal and self-absorption, irritability and depression, and a despairing malaise coupled with feelings of helplessness, pain, and unease. The only distinctive physical signs that belonged to her sleepless state were deep rings under her eyes, the slumping posture resulting from her exhaustion, and the deeply etched fatigue lines on her face.

Nicole awakened much too early, sometimes even in the middle of the night, and then was unable to fall back to sleep the rest of the night.

She seemed desperate, so I started active treatment with a low dosage sedating antidepressant during this initial visit, although I prefer to complete a workup that includes two weeks of sleep log entries before reaching a decision about the therapeutic approach. The effort taken in this case, though, proved successful. At the next visit, a smiling, alert, relaxed young woman stepped into my office—remarkably different in appearance, behavior, and attitude from the zombielike person who had presented herself at the first meeting.

Causes of Early A.M. Insomnia

Nicole's insomnia was triggered by a unique marital arrangement. She had been employed by an auction firm in France and was given the opportunity to assume an important position in New York. The appointment was one that she could not refuse, and the job was scheduled to last only a limited number of years. Since her husband, a university professor, could not easily give up his post to accompany her, a compromise was reached. Every month she would free herself from her duties and spend one week in Paris with him. Similarly, he would adjust his schedule so that he could spend one week each month in New York with her. In this way they were able to be together half of the time, despite their separation. The plan seemed to work, except that when she was in New York without him she suffered from seemingly implacable insomnia. When they were together, whether in New York or Paris, she was fine and slept well. It was during one of her severely distressing sleepless periods that she consulted me.

I make the assumption that an underlying depression is probably present in dealing with early morning insomnia. I use a consistent approach with all my cases of early A.M. insomnia, whether or not there are any immediately discernible circumstances that may be giving rise to a depression.

The most typical circumstance that brings about a depressive reaction is an emotional loss; a death or separation, a failed relationship, or a divorce. The loss of prestige, income, position, possessions, or even place or culture and group network can also cause depression.

The standard clinical symptoms of an overt depression are: an overwhelming sadness with feelings of loss; guilt and feelings of worthlessness and hopelessness; poor memory and concentration, the inability to make decisions, and irritability; social withdrawal and loss of interest and pleasure; and so-called vegetative signs. The last category includes bodily symptoms such as insomnia; loss of appetite, weight, or libido; constipation; or complaints of vague physical illnesses. Loss of energy and drive are frequent related features. Self-recriminations and self-blame are present in severe depressions and are often implicated in the development of self-destructive thoughts or actions. Depression, a very pervasive symptom in emotional difficulties, is present in a wide range of clinical pictures.

Various admixtures of complaints are found in the spectrum of the depressions. Young depressives usually present a brooding concern with problems of self-identity and self-confidence, associated with a generalized feeling of life confusion and nihilism. In contrast to older depressives, they generally show a sleep onset insomnia.

There is a mixture of both a depressed mood and a diffuse sense of anxiety and apprehension which doesn't seem to be fixated on any specific cause in some depressions.

There are masking attempts to cover up negative outlooks with pseudo-optimistic affirmative thoughts and behavior in the so-called "Smiling Depression." These depressives accentuate the affirmative! It is possible, with close observation, to penetrate this facade to find the passive, yet pervasive, pessimism lying underneath.

There is a strong dependency need in another depressive picture, with a tendency to cling and seek reassurance. There is also an opposite type that shows alienation, withdrawal, and defensiveness and wariness in social interactions. It is often found in an alienated rebellious young person.

Depressions may also be classified according to their origin, in addition to cataloging depressions by their clinical features. They are called "Reactive Depressions" if they result from a specific stress situation, usually a loss, or "Endogenous Depressions" if a biologic disposition is present and if attacks occur without any easily discernible external causes.

Sleep laboratory data have begun to show great promise in being able to differentiate the type of depression in difficult diagnoses. The findings that are emerging from this research are also being used theoretically to explain the origins of depressions.

Treatment of Early A.M. Insomnia

I treat early morning insomnia—if initial, nonspecific treatment modalities, like sleep hygiene, are ineffective—with exceedingly small amounts of sedating antidepressants. Doxepin and Desyrel are two that I commonly employ; they are obtainable by prescription only. The amount used is certainly not enough to act as an antidepressant in the usual clinical sense.

One of the speculative physiological theories advanced to explain depression is that it is linked to an interference with circadian

rhythm. I assume that the small quantity of antidepressant I pre-
scribe influences circadian rhythm in a way that restores the normal
sleep schedule that has been disrupted in the depression. Patients
remain on the antidepressant for approximately six weeks and then
are tapered off.

Early A.M. insomnia afflicts about ten to fifteen percent of my
patient population. I have been gratified by the success of my
method in practically one hundred percent of these patients. The
only exceptions which I have found in the many years since I began
this method are the following two cases.

In the first, though the diagnosis was confirmed by later sleep
laboratory followup, the patient did not respond to any attempts
at treatment at the laboratory, as far as I know. He worked on Wall
Street and had consulted me well before the 1987 crash; thus, his
condition was not related to that calamitous event. In my interviews
with him I suggested short term focal psychotherapy, after sedating
antidepressants failed to work, to see whether we could discover
the source of his intransigent insomnia. He declined, however, and
left treatment.

A curious footnote. Prior to October 1987 I had been seeing
many Wall Street people with insomnia. Surprisingly, after the
crash I had comparatively few referrals from that sector. I can only
speculate that stress, anchored in a real situation, might have something to do with short circuiting the development of neurotic com-
plexes. The grim reality of a sudden crash and lingering recession
is enough to worry about! A parallel phenomenon occurred during
the Blitz of London in World War II; the rate of neurosis declined,
presumably because reality stress diluted the individual emotional
conflicts of Londoners.

In my second case of early A.M. insomnia that did not initially
respond to the treatment technique, the results were far better. In
this instance Hortense Thomas, a young woman in her late twenties, was treated with focal psychotherapy when she did not respond to the usual regimen. Focal psychotherapy is short term
treatment, of approximately three to thirty sessions, focused
around the predominant complaint, in her case, insomnia, and con-
centrates on material which is primarily connected to the sleep
problem.

I found that Miss Thomas' sleep difficulties began when she was
faced with a specific decision. She is a research worker in a statis-

tical firm, and her department head, with whom she had a close working relationship, accepted a new position with a company in Washington, D.C. She was given the choice of accompanying him to the new location, or remaining in her job in New York under a new superior.

Her focus-oriented discussions with me revealed that a few years prior to this crisis she had been faced with another difficult choice that closely paralleled it. Her parents, who were Swiss, had been divorced and her mother remarried. After the second marriage, her mother, stepfather, and the children moved to the U.S. Her father later came to visit the family and on that occasion the patient was given the choice of living with her mother, stepfather, and the children or going to live with her father in Switzerland. After a great deal of emotional tension she decided to remain with her mother, and the matter was seemingly closed. However, the decision at her job reawakened reminiscences of the previous conflict that had not been fully resolved. This rerun led to a flareup of emotional problems that expressed themselves in the insomnia. When she was able to recognize this pattern and deal with it in her sessions with me, the insomnia cleared up, and her sleeping improved markedly.

She probably suffered from a "subclinical" depression, subclinical in the sense that, aside from the insomnia, there were no other depressive symptoms evidenced. This is often typical of mildly depressive states. Insomnia, though, is such an exquisitely sensitive indicator of emotional stress that it appears quite early in a wide array of psychological conflicts. Even in clearcut major depressions in which all the clinical symptoms, including insomnia, may have disappeared, polysomnography will often show the typical EEG sleep findings seen in depression. These EEG sleep findings indicate that a state of depressive vulnerability still exists in these patients, although otherwise they might be absolutely sunny in overt behavior and mood.

Other Causes of Early A.M. Insomnia

In dealing with early morning awakenings, care must be taken to rule out other causes that might be related to the symptom. The antidepressant technique is not effective in these circumstances, and treatment is primarily aimed at a correction of the underlying

basis of the difficulty. These other possibilities include environmental effects, such as the influence of light or noise. Many people,
highly sensitive to these stimuli, might be awakened by them in
the lighter portions of sleep during the wee hours.

REM sleep is frequent in this late sleep period. Medical phenomena that are often heightened during REM phases—ulcer-
caused pains, cardiac difficulties, or breathing problems associated
with lung and circulation problems, for example—should be
weighed as possible sources of an early A.M. insomnia. A sleep
upset may be the derivative of arthritic pains in this late, light
phase.

Other possible origins of early morning sleep difficulties include
temperature problems; and the shortening of sleep needs seen in
older people that often turns them into early birds who complain
of arising while the rest of the world sleeps on.

When the main complaint is insomnia but the clinical picture
shows a frank, major depression, treatment with an effective full-
scale antidepressant is used. This treatment is directed toward al-
leviation of the overt depression, not the insomnia. In fact, when
the medication relieves the depression, insomnia usually disappears.

The Long Term Antidepressant Problem

Antidepressant usage for melancholic conditions began in the late
1950s. Insomnia is a major symptom in depression, occurring in
more than ninety percent of cases.

There are instances where antidepressants successfully overcome clinical depression, only to have insomnia return when the
antidepressant is terminated. This new insomnia is not the result
of a reappearance of the depression, but is now being brought
about by worries about whether sleep will occur. The fear of being
unable to sleep has now created a "conditioned" insomnia markedly different in origin and nature from the prior, depression linked
sleeplessness. The problem is not early A.M. insomnia, but rather
unyielding sleep onset and middle insomnia, typical of conditioned
insomnia.

People with this form of insomnia immediately try to alleviate
the conditioned sleeplessness by resuming their now inappropriate
antidepressants. The use of antidepressants may be minimal at first,

but can increase to full strength, or even heavier, dosages. As a result, in recent years I've seen a number of persons who have been on large dosages of antidepressants for unusually long periods. I have known persons who have resorted to the use of antidepressants to combat their conditioned insomnias for periods as long as twenty-five years. It is a melancholy fact that antidepressants are relatively ineffective in conditioned insomnia, and barely touch the problem.

Sometimes these sufferers try to free themselves from their dependence on the antidepressants. This attempt is often done on a cold turkey basis and usually doesn't work. Even when withdrawal is gradual it is not successful. The persistent, intractable conditioned insomnia remains firmly in place, undercutting withdrawal from the drug since most persons give up and resume taking the medication when the loss of even the limited effects of the drug is felt.

Clinicians who deal with depression often seem ambivalent about this situation. On the one hand they feel that patients may be preventing not only the insomnia, but also the return outbreak of depression. They believe this long term treatment is justified, since the continued use of the antidepressant seems to have few deleterious effects.

These matters are especially relevant in the controversy over the long term usage of the newer antidepressants. They have such potent mood elevating and drive and energy enhancing properties, that even the general public clamors for them.

On the other hand, there is a strong feeling that such lengthy usage of a nonnatural chemical—with the possibility of the significant side effects seen with antidepressant use—may ultimately turn out to have severe negative effects, although they have not been demonstrated up to this point.

I use a long drug withdrawal program with a phased schedule that gradually substitutes placebos for the drug in dealing with this problem. This process takes about six months. It is not always effective because the conditioned insomnia pattern is reinforced in many cases by the person's rigid need to use sleeplessness as a repository of all anxiety. An onslaught of anxiety, which sometimes happens when there is even the most minimal sleeplessness in habit insomnia, makes these persons vulnerable to a fear that the insomnia will return. They then choose to go back to the seemingly harmless use of a partially successful medication, since the sedative side effect of the antidepressant may yield moderate benefits in aiding sleep.

Placing these long term antidepressant users in a support group treatment program, I find, can be helpful in freeing them from their drug dependency. Of course, the conditioned insomnia must also be treated with appropriate techniques. (These techniques are more fully presented in chapter 3, in Sleep Onset Insomnia.)

Seasonal Affective Disorder

A promising new technique for dealing with sleep timing problems like shift work, jet lag, and circadian disorders is called "Light Therapy" (exposure to very bright lights). This technique dates from 1980, when a research chemist first contacted the National Institute for Mental Health. He felt, as a chemist, that there was a relationship between the occurrence of his severe depressions and the winter season; that the absence of light at this time might play a role in his sleep and mood problems. The NIMH scientists, who had been working on the connection between bright light and the hormone melatonin (which is produced by the body at night and is tied to sleepiness), decided to test his assumption. He was treated with exposure to bright light, both mornings and evenings. Within three days his depression had lifted. A new and atypical form of depression had been identified and a treatment for it found. This hitherto overlooked type of depression was named "Seasonal Affective Disorder" and given the quite apropos acronym of SAD.

There has been a tidal wave of research on the use of light therapy as treatment for the winter seasonal forms of depression and a number of other conditions.

SAD involves symptoms beyond the usual ones shown by most depressions, and it has thus been designated an "Atypical Depression." There are a number of features of this depressive variant that are not shown in typical melancholias. They include difficulties in falling asleep, a tendency to delay lights-out time, excessive sleeping in the morning, weight gain, and a craving for carbohydrates.

Periodic, regularly recurring, serious winter depressions, occur in over 10 million Americans (six percent of the population) with a less severe variant—the "Winter Blues"—affecting another 25 million.

SAD tends to run in families. It crops up in children, where typical childhood symptoms like temper tantrums, cravings for junk foods, etc., make its symptom profile more covert and difficult to identify, except for its seasonal appearance. Women are more vulnerable to SAD than men. Most cases occur in persons in their twenties through forties.

The usual features of depression—sadness, lack of energy, withdrawal and work difficulties, decreased or absent sex drive, and even self-destructive tendencies—set in with the advent of winter. Along with these typical "rooted sorrows," as Shakespeare described melancholia, come a number of atypical symptoms that, surprisingly, are the reverse of those usually found in the depressions.

Rather than insomnia, there is hypersomnia (excessive sleeping), with SAD sufferers sleeping about an extra two and a half hours daily. They often have early bedtimes. More typically there is late morning awakening, oversleeping, and an excessive daytime sleepiness that leads to napping. An increase in nighttime waking, (middle) insomnia, and lighter restless sleep underlies the daytime sleepiness.

Also, in contrast to the typical depressive loss of appetite, there is an enormous craving for foods like carbohydrates, sweets, and heavy dishes like stews. These foods are usually soporific, but in SAD persons they seem to act as energizers, helping to keep SAD sufferers awake. Needless to say, this diet results in weight gain and the SAD-inflicted are always guilt ridden about their gluttony. An aching generalized anxiety, that torments the already overstressed SAD person, is also atypical for most other depressions. SAD women experience menstrual problems in the winters of their discontent.

Since the depressions of SAD are winter bound and a loss of libido accompanies their depressions, a consequence is that births in families where SAD exists tend to be concentrated in the late fall, since sex—like the Phoenix—arises in spring from the ashes of winter depressions.

This seasonal reawakening in spring and summer is the flip side of SAD. Previously burnt out, fatigued, sleepy, saddened persons undergo a remarkable renaissance when sunlight comes back into their lives.

Rather than merely returning to a normal baseline mood, many SAD persons are likely to go into overdrive in spring and summer, becoming almost manic. They have high energy; and are creative, optimistic, happy, and almost oversexed in these seasons. They sleep little, enjoy light foods, like salads, gobble up protein foods and fruits, are socially energetic, and are highly productive at work.

Summer Seasonal Affective Disorder

Contrary to the picture in SAD, there are also seasonal depressions which are linked to the summer season. Whereas periodic winter depressions are thought to be the result of the shortened period of daylight, the summer depressions are believed to be caused by excessive heat. Summer depressions do not respond to light therapy, however, and are more frequent than the winter variety, although the latter occur often enough. Summer seasonal depressions also show rebound in their "off season"—the winter—when manicky behavior is evident.

The summer seasonal depressions begin in May and end in September, whereas winter SAD begins in late October and ends in March.

Light Therapy—A New Nondrug Treatment

Exposure to very bright light in a directed program, using special fluorescent lamps, has been found to be effective as a treatment for winter SAD, as well as some other conditions. Light therapy treatment is used by the SAD sufferer throughout the winter months, when daylight is diminished.

Light therapy can be used alone or in conjunction with conventional treatment, using antidepressants. Light therapy alone, when effective, generally shows results after three or four days.

Light therapy does not work for summer SAD; only antidepressants are effective in the summer variety. Of course, a change of climate, like going to a warm sunny resort, will cure a northerner's winter seasonal depression or blues. Likewise, moving to a cool climate in the summer months will clear up the summer variety of SAD.

New advances in light therapy are procedural and technological. A recently developed tactic involves pinpointed light dosages that can adjust circadian rhythm problems. Even problems requiring as much as twelve hours of readjustment can be dealt with within three days.

The devices now being used and tested to provide light therapy often resemble Rube Goldberg oddities. They include visors of various design, eyeglass frame clipons, et al.

A new highly effective treatment for those winter blues is a dawn or dusk simulating device. Its rheostatic control regulates either a waxing or waning of light to simulate sunrise or sunset.

Light therapy was effective for one of my patients in correcting not only her morning wakeup problem and depression, but in eliminating her persistent weight control problem as well. Prior to its use she had been able to maintain a fairly rigid dietary discipline, except for a stubborn afternoon lust for carbohydrates. Carbohydrate craving, a major symptom of SAD, was particularly present in her case. Light therapy in the winter months succeeded in eliminating her afternoon dietary indiscretions and keeping her weight under control, as well as alleviating her morning wakeup difficulties and her disabling depression.

* * *

This light therapy vignette is a true story. A passenger wearing unusual glasses descended from a transatlantic flight that had just landed at Heathrow Airport outside London. Actually he was wearing welder's goggles, intended to shut out as much light as possible from his vision. This strange apparition was immediately surrounded by security conscious airport personnel and taken into custody for investigation. It turned out that he was an American sleep scientist who was applying what he had been learning about the newly recognized powerful influences of light as a cuing factor in biological rhythms in an attempt to deal with his jet lag!

Jet lag, shift work problems, premenstrual tension, and sleep disorders that involve inappropriate time shifts are other important conditions where the application of light therapy is being investigated.

* * *

When discussing light therapy, I must caution the reader that this procedure should be done only under the management of a sleep clinician.

A more detailed report on the topic of light therapy use is found in the Appendix.

Chapter 7

Mixed Types

Mixed types of insomnia, e.g., coexisting sleep onset and middle insomnias, are fairly common.

Pan-insomnia, the simultaneous occurrence of all three types, is much rarer.

The treatment strategy in the hybrid form is aimed at preventing a two-front war. The tactic is to focus on the type of insomnia associated with the greatest sleep difficulty, the one that serves as the main complaint. When this predominating insomnia is treated and overcome, the remaining problem usually clears up by itself. If not, then it is treated as called for by its own individuality.

These mixed types are not accidental, but are consequences of the nature of the underlying problems. For example, sleep onset insomnia is a result of high arousal at lights-out time. Often, once sleep has arrived after the initial sleep difficulty, the high arousal may be extinguished and a normal night may follow the sleep reluctance that was evident at bedtime. This may not always take place, and the sleeper may remain stirred up and unable to unwind completely. It follows that sleep will be lighter and more fragmented for the remainder of the night, and the ability to remain fully asleep may be blocked. The sleep disturbing arousal may gradually burn itself out over the course of the night, and the accumulated fatigue may be sufficient to grant an hour or so of sleep before dawn. At times, the arousal will become so intense that it lasts throughout the night, causing a pan-insomnia with zero sleep or, at most, a few intermittent, brief snatched moments of oblivion.

Another mixed pattern is seen with the parallel ocurrence of sleep onset and early A.M. insomnias. This twin insomnia can develop in a number of ways; for example, if poor sleep hygiene causes a sleep onset problem at the same time that a depression is creating early A.M. insomnia.

A further variation of this combination is caused by obsessive rumination patterns at the beginning of sleep, that go along with a depressive early A.M. sleep loss. My explanation for this particular pattern is that perfectionistic, obsessive individuals cannot let go of their defensive propensity for back and forth mental shifting, and tend to fall into a depression when their mental measures are not effective in containing a stressful situation. The obsessional arousal accounts for the sleep onset problem and the depression for the early A.M. difficulty. Low dosage sedating antidepressant treatment is of good use here, with the sedative properties of the antidepressant overcoming the initial sleep difficulties, and the antidepressant effects dealing with the early A.M. insomnia at the other end.

Kathy Kennedy, a young woman in her late twenties, consulted me about her insomnia. It had developed after the breakup of a romantic liaison. In the early course of treatment she showed a typical early A.M. insomnia that was successfully treated with a low dosage antidepressant. But, thereafter, whenever she was again in a romantic relationship that ended traumatically for her, she would respond with a reprise of her early morning insomnia. She decided to enter long term psychotherapy to deal with the conflicts that underlay her problem. We found that her failed relationships, reflecting her choice of partners of poor quality, were predominantly of a masochistic nature. With continued treatment, she was able to overcome her self-defeating patterns in love and became more discriminating in her amorous involvements.

She was surprised to discover one day that she had developed a completely different sleep problem. Instead of an early A.M. insomnia, she now had sleep onset difficulties. This dramatic change could be explained by the fact that she was now capable of attempting a healthier, more mature pattern of love. She was beginning to challenge her basically defensive masochism, and to find that her healthier new mode of relating did not automatically break up and end in painful loss. This change was disquieting, however, because it was so unfamiliar, causing a great deal of anxiety and ongoing arousal and resulting in the novel difficulty of falling asleep at bedtime. Treatment at this point was aimed at reducing her anxiety and giving her reassuring insight into the way her changed pattern of relating affected her sleep.

Kathy's treatment course showed a shifting pattern of insomnia, determined by the changed dynamics that were produced by the psychotherapeutic process.

An interesting case of mixed initial and middle insomnias was that of a retired, sixty-five-year-old sea captain. When first interviewed, he reported that he had undergone coronary bypass surgery for anginal pains about six years prior to seeing me. The operation relieved him of his anginal symptoms but he began to suffer from a severe insomnia, attributable to the stress of continuing financial difficulties that began at that time. His sleep logs showed a lights-out time of 9:30 P.M., protracted sleep onset insomnia, and a middle insomnia consisting of periods of wakefulness of an hour or two. Since he indulged in catchup sleep, his waketime was delayed until eight or 9 A.M. When he couldn't sleep during the night he would get out of bed and sit at a table in his living room, attempting to bring on sleep by resting his head on his arms on the table. When sleep didn't come this way, he would shift to the use of a couch or a contoured chair. Here he might sleep for a short time, and then switch back to the table, finally returning to the bed near dawn when he would succeed in falling asleep for a brief time.

In my treatment I gradually forced his lights-out time back to eleven thirty or 11 P.M., and advised him to be sure to awaken and get out of bed every morning at 6 A.M. However, it was clear after a short period of time that this treatment technique was not going to work. It resulted in some improvement, but the pattern of the insomnia was not sufficiently diminished to afford him relief from the next day's symptoms of fatigue and malaise.

Short term focused psychotherapy was begun. The interviews demonstrated an evident anxiety that focused on his cardiac status and on the economic situation in which he found himself. Reassurance about his medical situation and a demonstration of the high correlation between the economic stress and his sleep problems, as well as insightful help about the deeper sources of his anxiety, gradually increased his sleep capacity.

As the captain's coping ability increased he no longer had recourse to his tried and true method of getting out of bed to sit at his table in the living room for most of the night. This practice was traced to his habit, when he was an active sea captain, of sitting in his ward room when sailing dangerous waters, such as a close landfall. He was careful in these dangerous traverses always to be available instantly through his presence at the ward room table. With the advent of the physical and financial squalls that he experienced, he resumed this emergency nautical practice, now as a landlubber in his apartment. The navigational precautions which he practiced at sea were not sufficient in the new milieu, and he required the additional aids of good sleep hygiene, sleep restriction advice, and effective counseling to make his way through these new waters. He succeeded and was able to report eventually as follows, "I wish to thank you for treatment and guidance. I am once again sleeping nights—without drugs or vitamin/nutrients!" Self-help remedies had not been successful in his case. The vitamins had been advised by his nutrition conscious wife and he had been taking over-the-counter sleep nostrums as well.

Insomnia Crises

Sometimes, patients enter treatment in situations of intense crisis. They usually report being totally unable to sleep night after night, or achieving sleep for very short periods of only an hour or so late in the night when total fatigue finally has its effect.

The periods of extreme sleeplessness may go on for days and even weeks. These sleep victims are extremely anxious, even to the point of panic. They are so aroused that they are even unable to nap during the day despite major sleep loss. They have histories of repeatedly going to emergency rooms in hospitals, seeking relief but seldom finding it.

One young man, for example, came to me with a crisis insomnia caused by a promotion at work. The need to achieve in the new position was so anxiety provoking that it resulted in intense arousal and an acute sleeplessness, which had persisted for over a week before he was seen. He was highly agitated and reported heavy indulgence in alcohol in an attempt to sedate himself, but was still unable to get to sleep. The severe insomnia persisted after he stopped using alcohol at my insistence. Benzodiazepine hypnotics, even in higher dosage, did not help him. As is typical of many of these crisis insomnias, his vocational situation was highly compromised by his difficulties in functioning. This, coupled with a resulting fear of loss of job, fed back to increase an already excessive anxiety.

I was eventually able to find a means to diminish his arousal

through measured use of a barbiturate hypnotic plus frequent office visits. He was able to overcome his problem with the lessening
of anxiety about insomnia, plus intense focal psychotherapy.

I usually recommend that patients in crisis take a week or two
off from work in order to reduce performance–need stress. This
provides them with an opportunity to deal with sleep, as well as
time to search for the causal conflicts that might have played a role
in the development of the insomnia. In such crises, patients must
be seen frequently. Control of medication is very rigid because of
the danger of overuse, and supplies of drugs are minimal, limited
in amount and duration, and withdrawn when the insomnia is lessened. It is important to try to identify the essential conflicts that
are playing a causal role in the stress situation as soon as possible
and attempt to deal with them quickly in spite of the high anxiety
of the patient. In the young man's case, his insomnia was identified
as an anxiety generated by his rivalry with a competitive fellow
employee that harkened back to significant episodes in his history.

Fortunately, such crises are not too frequent an occurrence with
patients coming for insomnia treatment. The more usual clinical
picture is that of a fairly serious chronic sleep loss and not an
emergency crisis reaction.

Continuing therapeutic support is of prime importance in these
cases. It is imperative immediately to institute good sleep hygiene
parameters to hasten the return to, and the fixation of, an adequate
sleep schedule.

Sleep hygiene principles, presented fully in the next chapter, are
applicable in all insomnias across the board.

Chapter 8

Sleep Hygiene

Sleep hygiene is a collection of recommended guidelines that promote good sleep. Following the rules of good sleep hygiene avoids maladaptive sleep habits and is the first line of defense for the insomniac.

Sleep is regulated by the interaction of two factors: the amount of time spent awake since our last sleep, and the rhythmic pulsation of an internal clock which sets our wake–sleep schedule. Following the rules of sleep hygiene helps these two factors to work harmoniously, insuring good sleep and daytime alertness. Many sleep problems can, surprisingly, be traced to seemingly minor sleep hygiene transgressions which throw these factors off, causing insomnia.

Sleep hygiene guidelines should be followed as strictly as possible for an extended period when sleep problems exist, in order to realize their full benefits.

Sleep Schedule Regularity

A basic principle of sleep hygiene is regularity in lights-out time and waketime. For good sleepers, the time of going to bed or getting up usually makes little difference, but if you are an insomniac, a consistent sleep schedule is crucial. A regular sleep schedule makes your internal clock work better and will help guarantee ease in falling and remaining asleep.

The more significant transition between waking and sleeping takes place in the morning. When waking, we go from a horizontal position to a vertical position, and experience a sharp dark-to-light change that is reinforced by the stimulus of morning daylight. This is coupled with an upsurge of energy in preparation for the day's work. As a result, waking is a more distinctive pace setter for the biological clock than the less sharply defined way we fall asleep.

If you suffer from insomnia, going to bed at regular times on a seven-days-a-week schedule is ideal. This rule should be flexible for young people who date and socialize on midweek nights and weekends, as well as for socially active adults. I tell them to be sure to get to bed no more than an hour or two later on evenings out, whereas maintaining their regular waketime as much as possible.

It is best to go to bed when you are sleepy. This fixes a happy association between sleep and bed. If you find yourself unable to fall asleep within a reasonably short period of time, and are upset about lying in bed awake, give up the struggle and get out of bed until you feel sleepy again.

If you've had a sleepless night, you should avoid trying to get extra sleep the next night. One night of ordinary sleep is usually enough to overcome the negative effects from the previous night's sleep loss, since we sleep more efficiently on the makeup night.

A timing problem is created if you sleep late on weekends to catch up after a night on the town. This usually occurs on Sunday, when you try to go to bed at the regular hour. Since the time you spent awake on Sunday has been shortened by your catchup sleep in the morning—or there was too much sedentary activity, like watching TV football or tennis games, or just lying around—your sleep drive is lessened. Sleep on Sunday night then becomes more difficult and results in what is called "Sunday Night Insomnia," followed in turn by the half-asleep "Monday Morning Blahs."

Presleep Winddown

A good rule to follow is to give yourself adequate winddown time before retiring. Its importance is evident in the following two insomnia problems.

Frances Merrill was a mature, highly energetic woman who was on the go all day and throughout the evening. Her evenings were spent on the telephone with her children, relatives, and friends; chatting with them and solving their problems. Between phone calls, she would set up tomorrow's split second schedule and do work on household accounting or personal papers. These activities would continue nonstop until bedtime.

Paul Simon was in his first year of medical school and struggling to master the enormous workload of learning anatomy, physiology, and histology, and a vast compendium of related mind-bending material. He was an intense competitor, with high standards, enrolled in a stressful program. He came from a family of physicians and was expected to uphold the family achievement record. To accomplish this goal Paul studied well into the night, staying awake until the early hours of the morning, especially before frequently scheduled recitations and exams.

Frances and Paul had trouble falling asleep and awoke many times during the night, finding it difficult—owing to their heightened arousal—to fall back to sleep. Their sleeplessness caused their daytime performances to suffer, and they consulted me about their insomnia. In both cases I advised them to eliminate as much evening presleep stress as possible. Frances was counseled to tell her friends and relatives not to call after an hour and a half before her lights-out time. Paul was told to drop his intense studying before sleep. Enjoying a period of rest and rehabilitation after the battles of the day enabled them to overcome their insomnia quickly.

Relaxing for at least an hour before bedtime should include enjoyable, winding down practices, such as reading or hobbies, which lower the arousal level. Many people use a warm bath or shower to relax at this time. Scheduling presleep relaxation before bedtime is a cardinal sleep hygiene principle.

Avoiding stress inducing situations during the period before going to bed is part of the presleep winddown. For example, this time should not be used for disciplining children. Consideration of other stressful matters should be left for a more propitious time. Staying away from absorbing mysteries and best-sellers before sleep is also a good idea.

Presleep Rituals

Presleep rituals are a comfort and help extinguish a lingering daytime arousal. Their soporific effects help smooth our way for relaxation and sleep. Opening windows, adjusting covers and pillows, brushing teeth, and a myriad of other automatic acts we repeat nightly are examples of sleep associated rituals. One of the important rituals necessary for some people is a safety check. This includes examining door locks and lights, making sure that any burglar alarms are working, and that the telephone is nearby for emergency use.

Napping

If you suffer from sleeplessness, you should try to avoid napping during the day. Sleep has been compared to a bank account. If you overdraw by napping during the day, you pay the piper by sleeping less that night to make up for the squandering of the reserve. The accumulation of fatigue during the day has been lessened by the nap. It lowers the sleep pressure level and the ability to fall asleep that night. If the urge to nap comes upon you during the day and seems irresistible, schedule things to do at those times, especially activities that require large body movements or those which absorb your total attention. If you need to overcome an overwhelming desire to nap close to bedtime, get up and walk around, wash your face with cold water, do calisthenics, write letters, make shopping lists, converse, or telephone someone. Playing loud, rapid music with vigorous rhythms or turning on bright lights are other arousing stimuli you might try.

There is some controversy about the practice of napping. Is it always detrimental to your ability to sleep well that night? To answer this question for yourself, take a nap in the afternoon. If your nap is followed by grogginess or poor sleep that night, then it is advisable for you to avoid napping.

The length of naps is also important. A study found that a nap of forty-two minutes is best to restore performance efficiency, but naps of lesser or longer duration may help, depending on the individual case.

Bed and Bedroom

What about the bed? Obviously, it must be large enough for comfort. A six-foot-two individual who sleeps on his side with knees drawn up, may be just as comfortable in a normal-sized bed as another person several inches shorter who sleeps stretched out on his back. A simple rule about bed size is to have enough room to turn over and move around comfortably without having the bed sway. In fact, among all the patients I have treated for insomnia, only one woman ever complained about her bed as a possible source of her problem, and even in this case I was dubious about the bed being the real difficulty!

There are any number of accessories to choose from in our search for comfortable and relaxing sleep, from extra layers of foam to mattresses that can be positioned at various angles, like hospital beds. A recent innovation is the use of eggcrate-like foam sheeting over the mattress. Its use is supposed to reduce pressure pain in those, like the elderly, who are susceptible. There are people who like very hard beds, or very soft beds; some like one pillow, or two, or even three pillows. Enrico Caruso, the great opera singer, slept on seventeen. Perhaps he needed them to reach high C. In any case, the features of your bed are something you can sort out for yourself.

If you live in a studio apartment without a separate bedroom, other areas of the room should be set aside for activities not related to sleep, and a room divider can be used to separate the bed from other space.

Crowding is an environmental factor that can be detrimental. Sometimes many people are forced to live and sleep in close proximity to one another, a common occurrence today when apartments are shared to reduce expenses. The different time schedules of the roommates can cause unwelcome noise, light, and other intrusive interruptions to rest and sleep. This happened to Allen and George, who shared a large apartment with three bedrooms. To help defray expenses they invited Larry to sublet the third bedroom. This arrangement had its pecuniary advantages for Allen, but it also created some disadvantages. Allen suffered from chronic insomnia and, in an attempt to overcome his sleep problem, decided to adhere very strictly to sleep hygiene rules. He therefore shut his door about an hour and a half before bedtime and tried to achieve relaxation through reading and other tranquilizing activities.

The new roommate, Larry, was gregarious and looked to Allen as a social mentor. He often knocked on Allen's closed door, interrupting Allen's attempt at solitude and sleep prophylaxis. A very polite and somewhat inhibited person, Allen was hesitant to complain about the intrusions. He was eventually able to overcome his scruples, and to tactfully confront Larry about the problem and end the disruption with counseling, however. He got rid of a large impediment which had prevented him from following the rules of sleep hygiene. This eventually enabled him to overcome his insomnia.

Bed, Bedroom, and Sex

It is a good sleep hygiene rule to restrict the use of the bed solely to sleep and to sex. If, instead of being relaxing, sex is experienced as arousing in the postcoital period, it should be left for hours other than those for sleeping; if this is not possible, it should be transferred to another setting in the house.

All activities aside from sleep and sex should be banished from the bedroom and take place in other areas in the house. Bed and bedroom should not be used for telephone conversations, watching TV, listening to music, or watching videos. Eating in bed, working, or writing letters there, or even resting during evening or presleep hours, are all taboo. Radios and CDs are also forbidden. These measures help to avoid linking the bedroom with arousal and making sleep more difficult to come by at bedtime.

Temperature, Light, Humidity, and Noise

Our body temperature is high during the day and begins to dip about two hours prior to normal bedtime. It reaches its lowest point around 5 A.M., when it begins to rise again. The dip reflects the body's slowdown and is the reason we like to be cool at bedtime. We prefer warmth at waketime to parallel the energizing rise in body temperature which occurs in the morning.

Temperatures between sixty-four and sixty-eight degrees Fahrenheit seem to be best for sleep. Too high a temperature is worse for you than one that is too low, and temperatures above seventy degrees may result in frequent awakenings and restlessness. For this reason sleep is more difficult in the summer than in the winter months. In these days of universal air conditioning, though, this problem is minimized. However, if your bedroom is too cold your sleep will become disrupted by shivering as your body attempts to generate more heat. For some reason, this is associated with dreams that have nightmarish qualities. If you suffer from cold feet at night that disturbs sleep, you could try wearing socks or using a hot water bottle.

Humidity, like temperature, has implications for sleep comfort. If you find you cannot sleep in a room that is too dry, it may be because it gives you a scratchy throat and stuffed-up nose. Humidifiers can alleviate dryness and give you relief. Too much humidity, on the other hand, will make you sweaty and uncomfortable.

Eighty percent of our incoming sensory information is delivered visually by means of light. Some individuals are very sensitive to light. If this troubles you and the unwelcome effects of light at night prevent "shut-eye," a sleep mask is recommended. Blackout curtains are also sometimes necessary. Dark tones in your bedroom furnishings, and color schemes that absorb light can help, too.

Noise is a significant disturber of sleep. Many people, sensitive to sound, awaken at the slightest whisper; others can sleep through explosions. Sound sense acts like sonar equipment on submarines. It protects us during sleep, when the nervous system is constantly on the alert to possible danger coming our way.

We do not have to be fully awake to suffer the ill effects of noise disturbance. Even though we are not fully awake, noise may cause an increase in both "microawakenings" and lightening of sleep that is enough to be followed by next day drowsiness and other unpleasant consequences. When a regularly recurrent noise does not portend danger, it no longer disturbs our sleep. Intermittent sounds, on the other hand, always catch us off guard and are disturbing and difficult to endure.

People exposed to noises that interfere with sleep use various tactics to screen them out. Some insomniacs use earplugs, noise-abating curtains and carpets, soundproofing materials to insulate the bedroom, double-paned windows, white sound machines, fans and air conditioners, radios, and other auditory defenses.

Fluid Restriction

Fluid intake should be restricted prior to sleep, avoiding the necessity of waking to urinate during the night, a practice which might give you trouble falling back to sleep. If you feel dry and need fluids at bedtime or during the night, the amount you drink should be limited. Small sips of milk, fruit juice, or preferably, water, are recommended. This caveat is especially important for seniors, who normally have lightened sleep.

Exercise

It had been thought that exercise during the day increased the ability to enjoy more of the deep phases of sleep. This has been found to be false, except in the case of trained athletes.

If you find that exercise helps you relax, it should be done at least six hours before bedtime. Too close to lights-out time will be arousing and, therefore, counterproductive.

Hydrotherapy

A hot bath two hours prior to sleep will cause a cooling effect that can help bring on sleep. Bringing down the body temperature in this way helps induce drowsiness. A caveat here is that this technique should not be practiced by pregnant women.

Diet

Diet is very significant in relation to sleep. In late evening meals, avoid foods that are heavy and greasy, since they may cause sleep-disruptive digestive discomfort. Foods that are gas producing or spicy and acidic might give rise to heartburn or other distress, and you should not indulge in them too close to bedtime. It takes about two and a half hours to clear the stomach of food; this should be your guide to when you eat your last meal. Although this rule may be difficult to follow in our modern urban society, where it has become customary to dine late in arousing circumstances, the sleep seeker should avoid eating too near retiring.

Certain foods are thought to help sleep. Some experts recommend light carbohydrate snacks or carbohydrate and milk combinations at bedtime. Carbohydrates in the form of toast, English muffins with jam, graham crackers, marshmallows, or pasta have been reported to be helpful in inducing sleep. However, if you are calorie conscious, try to reduce the amount in your evening meal to compensate for the increased intake at bedtime.

It is not advisable to snack if you awaken and can't fall back to sleep. This is a common misstep. By satisfying a craving to eat at this time, you reinforce a night feeding schedule. The clever body will then wake up, like Pavlov's dog, in anticipation of the oral gratification to come, increasing the likelihood of sleep loss. You should not feed this habit. Eating is a strict no-no during the night. Insomniacs, stay out of the kitchen!

People who have major eating problems, like bulimia or anorexia, have some special handicaps in addition to the sleep difficulties directly caused by the eating disorder. Frequently, they are covert about their problem in their behavior. For example, a young woman patient had been going with a man to whom she eventually became engaged. Their dating pattern was to spend weekends together in his apartment. During the week she slept at home in her parents' house. She suffered from bulimia but didn't want her fiance to become aware of it. When staying overnight at his apartment she would wait until he fell asleep and then creep out of the bedroom, slink down to the kitchen, and gorge. When living with her parents, who knew about her problem, she would also be seized at night by the insatiable need to eat. But in her own home she could awaken and go down to the kitchen to indulge in a feeding frenzy without fear. In both situations, however, her sleep suffered. I successfully treated her sleep disruption with a program of strict sleep hygiene, and referred her to an eating disorders program, where she was finally able to deal with her bulimia.

Caffeine

Caffeine, a nervous system stimulant, is often a cause of insomnia. It is present in coffee, tea, cocoa, chocolate, and a variety of medications, both those obtained by prescription and over-the-counter. Restricting or eliminating the use of caffeine is a major sleep hygiene guideline.

The usual source of caffeine in our diets is coffee. Americans use one-third of the coffee consumed in the world. The average coffee drinker has three and a half cups a day. Some insomnia victims use coffee during the day to overcome the loss of vitality caused by poor sleep. The dangers of coffee lie in either overdoing it by drinking too much during the day, or by having it too close to bedtime. The stimulant effects of coffee are evident after two successive cups. The average cup of coffee contains between 100 and 150 milligrams (mg) of caffeine. Caffeine reaches its peak level in blood about one hour after ingestion and achieves its maximum effectiveness within two to three hours.

People vary in their sensitivity to coffee. Half of those who drink coffee find that it interferes with their sleep when taken near bedtime, whereas the other half report no subjective feelings of sleep influence. Paradoxically, coffee at bedtime may help you sleep if your body is aroused by the withdrawal effect of not having had any caffeine for quite a while. Drinking coffee in these circumstances quiets the withdrawal effect, and dissipates the headaches, depression, lethargy, and sleeplessness that go with it. Headaches during the afternoon and evening may be a withdrawal sign if you drank a lot of coffee at breakfast or lunch.

Coffee works in the body by blocking adenosine, a neural transmitter that inhibits nervous activity. This, in turn, results in the experience of arousal. Coffee's effects can last from eight to fourteen hours in people who are sensitive to caffeine. A single cup of coffee in the morning, if you are a caffeine sensitive person, can interfere with your sleep that night, causing an increased number of awakenings, difficulty in falling asleep, and a decrease in total sleep amount. No matter how little coffee you take during the day, if you have sleep difficulties, it is advisable to forgo any coffee, or caffeine-containing beverages or foods, within six hours of bedtime. As a practical measure, coffee should not be ingested by insomnia sufferers—even in minimal or moderate amounts—after the noon hour. To discover your sensitivity to caffeine, eliminate all sources for one week and then check to see if abstinence makes you feel better.

Brewed coffee contains the most caffeine, instant coffee the least. Tea has less caffeine, averaging between 50 and 100 mg a cup, and green tea has less than black tea. A glass of most cola drinks contains about 50 mg of caffeine. (The caffeine that is extracted from coffee in making decaffeinated coffee is used by the soft drink industry to produce their beverages.) Cocoa contains about 15 mg of caffeine a cup. Pure milk chocolate contains about 15 mg an ounce. The average chocolate bar, therefore, contains about 25 to 50 mg of caffeine.

Some commonly used drugs contain caffeine. Excedrin, the pain killer, contains 65 mg, Empirin Compound has 32 mg, Anacin has 32 mg, and Dristan has 16 mg; other cold and allergy remedies also contain significant amounts. Midol, used to relieve menstrual difficulties, contains 32 mg a tablet. Prescription drugs such as Darvon Compound (35 mg), Diuril, a diuretic (40 mg), and migraine medications usually contain significant amounts. You should always check the contents of over-the-counter medications to ascertain whether caffeine is contained in the product.

If you have sleep difficulties, check with your physician about the stimulating effects of the medications prescribed for you. Decongestants can contain stimulants, as can drugs that combat obesity. Steroids, thyroid drugs, and a host of other pharmaceuticals have significant stimulant effects. If it is necessary to use such drugs, your doctor might consider decreasing the amount or switching you to another drug without stimulating effects.

Nasal sprays are often used prior to sleep to get rid of stuffiness that interferes with sleep. This habit has hidden pitfalls. These sprays contain stimulants which cause arousal and actually may contribute to sleep difficulties. If you are using sprays and experiencing sleep problems, you should check with your doctor, who can advise you on the availability of other sprays which do not have sleep-disruptive qualities.

Alcohol

In contrast to caffeine, alcohol is a central nervous system depressant. Insomniacs frequently resort to the use of alcohol as a sleep aid. The danger with this lies in three directions. First, even though it helps us to fall asleep, the soporific effect of alcohol is lost later when the alcohol is metabolized, to be followed by arousing withdrawal effects. This may initiate an insidious cycle if heavier indulgence is tried in attempting to overcome the sleep disturbing withdrawal effects. Increasing amounts of alcohol can lead to eventual dependence and abuse. An early evening cocktail, though, helps us to relax and leaves enough time for metabolism of the alcohol to take place without disturbing sleep. A drink or two taken as a nightcap before bedtime, though, may ruin your sleep.

The second danger is perspiration. The drop in body temperature which accompanies sweating can help bring on sleep, since cooling at bedtime fosters slumber. The problem occurs later. Alcohol begins to be metabolized by the body in the relatively brief time of approximately one hour. With metabolism, the sleep inducing effect of sweating is lost. An opposite arousing reaction takes place, caused by withdrawal, which produces a restless sleep riddled with many awakenings. The withdrawal effects, once started, can persist for hours, even after the blood alcohol is totally eliminated.

The third danger is that alcohol causes suppression of REM. When alcohol wears off, REM rebounds under pressure. The REM rebound manifests itself in bizarre, frightening dreams that cause restlessness, agitation, poor sleep, or actual awakening.

In habitually heavy drinkers, the effects are even more intense. Sleep is interrupted and broken into several nonrefreshing segments. The effects on brain physiology in the heavy drinker are quite marked. Even after withdrawal from alcohol and regained sobriety, abnormal EEG rhythm patterns can last for months or years—or even a lifetime. These abnormal rhythms are linked to disturbed sleep, and consequent daytime inefficiency and mood problems.

Poor sleepers over the age of fifty should be doubly cautious about using alcohol as a nightcap. There is an increased tendency to experience breathing difficulties during sleep at this age. Alcohol is sedating and its combination with the already compromised respiration that accompanies a sleep apnea, when present, may result in dire consequences.

"Which came first?" is often the question when sleep and alcohol problems coexist. Did the insomnia cause excess drinking or did the alcohol abuse predate the sleep problem? To help answer this puzzle we must ask whether the drinking is restricted to the presleep period, or if getting to sleep was the original problem. Other relevant questions are whether life problems are present for the drinker (apart from the insomnia) and whether the motivation exists to stop using alcohol to solve a sleep difficulty.

Nicotine

Turning to another common drug that frequently causes sleep problems, beware of the fact that nicotine is a stimulant. Nicotine causes the release of epinephrine, a central nervous system energizer. At low levels of epinephrine there is mild euphoria, an effect produced in moderate smokers. For heavy smokers the effect is arousal. Since withdrawal from nicotine does not begin until two to three hours after smoking, effects on sleep are varied, depending somewhat on the concentration of nicotine and the time of smoking. The mild smoker may smoke at bedtime and feel relaxed enough to fall asleep, but then the stimulating effects might make themselves felt later and be arousing enough to cause awakening. This is further compounded by the occurrence of withdrawal during even later stages of sleep.

It takes smokers, even moderate ones, an average of fourteen minutes longer than nonsmokers to fall asleep; and smokers awaken more frequently during the night than do nonsmokers.

The concurrent use of nicotine and alcohol intensifies these effects. A young woman smoker who consulted me had a difficult time getting to sleep and fell into the habit of using wine to assist her sleep search. Treatment uncovered that her coinciding use of cigarette smoking and wine drinking at bedtime accounted for her insomnia problem. The insomnia disappeared when she stopped smoking and discontinued the use of wine as a sleep potion.

Most smokers refrain while hospitalized. I have treated some smokers who tried to continue their abstinence after hospitalization, believing they were halfway home in breaking their cigarette habit. Sadly, however, the cold turkey hospital withdrawal schedule usually causes insomnia. This onset of insomnia made my patients so anxious that even after the withdrawal effects subsided, their traumatic experience of sleep anxiety resulted in outbreaks of a conditioned insomnia that plagued them. They failed to realize that it was the conditioning process and not the nicotine withdrawal, as they had believed, that was causing their protracted insomnia. Pointing this out helped them accept the insomnia deconditioning program that eventually freed them of the problem.

Sleep Hygiene Guidelines Summary

1. Keep regular times of going to sleep and waking, seven days a week.
2. Go to bed only when sleepy, but be sure to get up at your regular waketime. Remember, waketime is more important than lights-out time in regulating sleep.
3. If you must go to bed later once or twice a week, do not remain awake longer than an hour (or at most two) past your regular bedtime. Sleep late on the weekend (preferably on the first

day of the weekend), if necessary, to make up for sleep lost during the week. In any case, do not go over the limit of an hour or two in a day for the amount of your catchup sleep.

4. Give yourself an hour or two of winddown time before going to bed.
   a. Do things that are not arousing and that relax you.
   b. Use the bed only for sleep and sex. If sex is too arousing and interferes with sleep, schedule it for another time or in another place if possible.
   c. Learn to associate the bed and bedroom only with sleep.
   d. Do not watch TV, do bills or other paperwork, listen to the radio, eat, etc. in the bed.
   e. Read in bed only if it is a brief part of your presleep ritual and does not involve absorbing reading matter that you cannot put down.

5. Have a regular presleep routine. Establish it as a ritual that is associated with sleep and security. Wash, brush teeth, void bladder, set temperature, lay out next day's clothing, do a lock check, etc., in the same order every night.

6. Make sure your bedroom is conducive to sleep.
   a. Avoid too hot or too cold a bedroom temperature.
   b. Minimize sound. Use a white sound machine or earplugs to block out noises that disrupt sleep.
   c. Use a sleep mask or blackout curtains to eliminate light.
   d. Make sure your bed is large enough and has the right mattress, pillows, and covers to be comfortable.
   e. Wear loose clothing (if you do not sleep in the nude).
   f. Have bedroom fixtures and decorating schemes that are compatible with your personality and that relax you.

7. Avoid stress, worry, and arguments before going to bed. (See chapter 9 on relaxation methods.)

8. Do not clock watch. Use alarms to awaken in the morning. Put them under the bed, facing away from you, or in a drawer. Use a backup alarm or commission a family member or bed partner to awaken you, if this is necessary.

9. Avoid too much caffeine during the day and abstain from coffee or caffeine containing beverages or food for at least six hours before bedtime (or even better, from noon on).

10. Avoid other arousing substances, like drugs that are stimulating, e.g., asthma remedies, diet drugs, steroids and similar bio-

logical excitants, and nose drops (most contain arousing ingre-
dients). If it is necessary to use these medications, check with
your doctor on the minimum dosage possible or on substitute
nonstimulating medication.

11. Alcohol should not be used as a nightcap, or taken for at least
four hours before bedtime.

12. Avoid use of nicotine at bedtime if you smoke, as it is arousing.

13. Avoid heavy meals or spicy or gas producing foods too close to
bedtime. A light carbohydrate snack or light dairy food at bedtime helps to induce sleep. Do not snack during the night. If
you are thirsty take only a few sips of water or fruit juice.

14. Avoid drinking too much fluid before sleep. The resulting need
to go to the bathroom may awaken you and the arousal can
cause difficulty in getting back to sleep.

Chapter 9

Relaxation Techniques

When adherence to sleep hygiene guidelines for a sufficient length of time fails to overcome a sleep problem, use of effective relaxation techniques may do the trick. Relaxation techniques are effective when tension, especially tension owing to muscle strain, prevents sleep, or when worrying and the inability to turn the mind off causes insomnia. Mark Twain had a very simple solution to these problems. He said, "When I can't sleep I simply move to the side of the bed and then fall off." The chronic insomniac needs more practical advice.

You must be mentally and physically relaxed to fall asleep, unless you are so tired that simply assuming a horizontal position is enough to induce slumber. Relaxation is the entrance hall to the castle of sleep. The relaxed brain is characterized by the production of "alpha" waves. The prerequisite for sleep is achievement of the alpha state, resting quietly with eyes closed. It is relatively simple to "fall off" into slumber from this state. Practitioners of yoga, who devote themselves to the achievement of an alpha state, often find it a difficult task to prevent themselves from going all the way and falling asleep.

The largest single enemy of the ability to fall asleep is the state of arousal caused by what I call the worry machine. I liken the tendency to ruminate when trying to fall asleep, or the continual intrusion of worries from the day world into the bedroom, to a magnet that compellingly draws our thoughts to a stressful or arousing pitch and prevents alpha. The aim of a relaxation program is to neutralize the magnetic action of this worry machine. Frequently heard comments of insomniacs are, "I can't turn my mind off," or "the minute I get into bed I start worrying," or "I'm not relaxed, I can't fall asleep." In a survey, one-third of people with insomnia reported that their difficulty was caused by "thinking over" their problems. Twenty-five percent said they couldn't sleep because of an inability to relax, and eleven percent could not sleep because they were overstimulated. Only very rarely do I get patients who say they cannot fall asleep and just do not have anything on their minds to account for this difficulty.

The usual sources of worry are personal and emotional problems, job difficulties, and health concerns. Worrying seems to be at its peak during the presleep period when the distractions of daytime activity are absent. Relaxation exercises are aimed at undoing this focus on worry. Yet how difficult it is! No matter how hard the attempt to deflect attention, the wayward mind always seems to snap back to the worry magnet. Since we cannot deal with the existing stress itself in an actual active way while we're lying in bed, we must do it in the substitute form of thinking, a less direct and more tenuous modality.

This inadequacy and the resulting frustration account for the intensity of the struggle. When the worry is strong and serious, or when there is a built-in psychological tendency to conquer problems with thinking, or when the sleep situation in itself is somewhat threatening, then the goal of sleep relaxation can only be attained with some degree of difficulty. The sleep relaxation exercises that follow have been devised to deliver the slumber seeker from this quandary. They merit trial and can work.

Breath Control

Sleep enhancing breathing exercises are simple yet effective techniques of relaxation. Good singers are often good sleepers because they have mastered the elements of breath control. When we fall asleep a number of integrated bodily processes automatically slow down. Temperature declines, the pulse rate slows, blood pressure falls, and breathing slows down and diminishes in amplitude. Slowing breathing by itself is an effective way of initiating this process, causing the state of arousal to decelerate and go into the low gear characteristic of sleep. This deceleration will automatically usher in the onset of alpha.

Here are eight breathing exercises that can be effective:

1. The technique known as the Relaxation Response utilizes these principles. In the relaxation response, one takes a deep breath, holds it, and breathes out slowly, protractedly saying "one" at the same time to prolong the exhalation. This is repeated a number of times in order to produce a relaxed state.

Another good way to slow breathing is to breathe in and out through your nostrils. To do this, one must "zip the lips," and exhale and inhale only through the nose.

2. Take a deep breath through the nose, hold it while counting mentally to ten, then exhale as slowly as possible. A variant of this exercise is to inhale to the count of three, exhale to the count of three, and then hold your breath as long as possible. Repeat five to eight times.

3. A yoga technique involves alternate breathing through right and left nostrils. Press the right thumb to close the right nostril; inhale to the count of five slowly; close the left nostril with the second or third finger; release the thumb and exhale slowly to the count of ten. Then inhale through the right nostril for a count of five; close the right nostril with the thumb; release the left nostril from the finger and exhale through the left for a count of ten. The time of alternately inhaling and exhaling might be increased slowly, maintaining the proportion of exhalation to inhalation of two to one.

4. Lie with your arms at your sides and breathe in slowly through the nose and then out through the mouth. Follow this procedure by inhaling with your mouth open; at the end of the indrawn breath, yawn as widely as possible. Repeat this procedure.

5. While lying down, slowly raise your head and upper parts of your body while exhaling, then lower your head and upper body while slowly inhaling. A variation of this exercise involves use of the legs. Lying on your back, lift one leg about halfway up, to forty-five degrees, while exhaling; then lower the leg while slowly inhaling. Repeat the process with the other leg.

6. Place a moderately heavy book on your stomach and try to push it as high as possible while exhaling through the nose. Then have it sink as deeply as possible while inhaling slowly through the nose.

7. Lie on your back with your hands and arms at your sides. Stretch out full length, and then breathe in slowly and deeply, raising your arms over your head while pressing with your body

against the bed. Hold your breath for a count of ten and stretch your body as much as possible. Exhale slowly and while doing so bring your arms slowly back again to the original position.

8. Lie down with your hands placed at the margin of your ribs and abdomen. Pressing down with your hands, breathe in through your nose to a count of five. Hold your breath for one count, and then let your breath out slowly for a count of five; at the same time, slowly loosen the pressure of your hands on the rib-abdominal margin.

Any number of these breathing exercises may be done in combination with the others. They may be repeated for a number of times to reach a state of relaxation.

Yawning, Snoring, Sighing

Before leaving the topic of breathing and respiration in relation to sleep, we should take note of two interesting and important phenomena: yawning and snoring. Yawning and snoring are in a sense opposites. Yawning is a phenomenon occurring during wakefulness, and snoring takes place during sleep; we are conscious while yawning, but we have no memory of snoring since we are asleep. In yawning the mouth is opened widely, and the tongue and back of the tongue move forward. All the jaw muscles are contracted and tight. In snoring, on the other hand, the base of the tongue falls back against the back wall of the throat and the muscles of the mouth and throat are lax.

We have no definitive reasons for the function and mechanisms of yawning. Yawning, which takes place in animals as well as in humans, is initiated by boredom, fatigue, and sleepiness as well as by mimetic tendencies. Seeing someone else stretch and yawn induces like behavior. Until recently it was believed that yawning was initiated by a lowered oxygen level in the blood and was an attempt to gulp in large amounts of air to replenish this loss. But newer evidence has disproved this theory. Yawning is now thought of as an arousal defense reflex. The deep inhalation of breath facilitates blood flow and results in more oxygen being available for an increased metabolic rate. The body is stimulated by contraction of the diaphragm and stretching of the limbs, which stimulates the muscles of the rib cage, arms, mouth, and jaw to also tighten. The stimulation caused by this action triggers an arousal. Paradoxically, such arousal is followed by a state of tranquility and a lowered level of arousal as the muscles relax after clenching. However, yawning does not lead to sleep. It leads to waking, and it usually occurs before bedtime and on waking up.

Snoring is the term for sounds produced by the partial obstruction of breathing in sleep. It has a high incidence, being found in twenty percent of men and five percent of women in the thirty- to thirty-five-year-old age group. This difference is a result of the differences in fat distribution in the throats of men and women. Snoring increases with age, so that at sixty years of age, sixty percent of men and forty percent of women snore. The increase in the incidence of snoring in women in the later years is a result of the loss of tone of the throat musculature. The female sex hormones that previously maintained the tone are lost after menopause.

Snoring does not occur in most animals. Animals sleep prone or on the side and this prevents the jaw and base of the tongue from falling back against the wall of the throat.

Most remedies for snoring are designed to move the sleeper from the supine (face upward) position, or to position the lower jaw and base of the tongue forward, or to arouse the sleeper. Snoring can be a serious familial and social problem. The most significant aspect of snoring, aside from its household sleep disruption, is its occurrence as part of the obstructive sleep apnea disorder, when breathing actually fully stops for a time and then abruptly starts again. The mechanism of snoring is a vibration of the soft palate and the walls of the throat by air passing over them.

Here are some remedies for the snoring problem.

Lose weight.
Have an examination by an ear, nose, and throat doctor.
Limit or discontinue a smoking problem.
Sew a pocket to the back of pajamas, and place a ball there.
Elevate head of the bed, or use extra pillows to sleep high.
Wear a surgical collar to bed.

For the sleep partner:
Wear earplugs.
Use white sound machine to muffle snores.
Get larger bed or use separate beds or bedrooms.

See chapter 12 under Sleep Apnea for other techniques.

A nighttime breathing phenomenon that is a cousin of yawning and snoring is sighing. Sighing is caused by taking deep breaths to expand the lungs. This process normally occurs between one and twenty-five times per night, and tends to take place in episodes of two sighs at a time.

Early Warning Signs of Sleep

The onset of the state of sleepiness is recognized by the signal of a slight yawn. The eyelids become droopy, with a sense of the need to rub them because of the accumulation of sealing mucus. These signs are accompanied by a delicious sense of muscular relaxation and the tendency to stretch.

It is most important to be on the lookout for these early warning signs of impending sleepiness. If you are out of bed you must make tracks without delay and return to bed, settling comfortably into your preferred sleep position for falling asleep—whether it's on the side, facedown, or on the back.

If you are in bed when the premonitory signs of sleepiness occur, and if you are not a back sleeper, immediately turn to your preferred sleep position in the bed, whether it's on your side, facedown, or whatever. Most people know their preferred position for falling asleep (see chapter 15) and can utilize this knowledge with the techniques described.

It is especially important not to disregard the early warning signs of sleepiness. It is a mistake to think that waiting for increased manifestations of these signs will yield a more intense feeling of sleepiness. If this mistake is made, what usually happens is an overshoot into an alerted state. Overlooking these early signs is most likely followed by a reflex arousal; once in this state, it will take longer to retrace the steps to the lost Utopia of impending sleep.

While properly heeding the early warning signs and assuming the preferred sleep position, continue the relaxation exercises that resulted in yielding sleepiness, repeating them if necessary, as well as continuing to breathe in and out through the nose. These procedures should lead to sleep.

Relaxation Exercises

All of the relaxation exercises to be described in the following pages can be done either in or out of bed. When relaxation exercises are performed in bed, lie comfortably on your back with hands resting at your sides, or on your lower abdomen. If the exercises are done out of bed, on a couch or on the floor, your body position should again be supine—on your back with hands and arms resting comfortably at your sides. A recliner may be used if available. Even a comfortable chair will do.

When should you stay in bed and when should you get out of bed and go to another location? This depends to a large extent on whether you can remain relaxed and at ease in bed, despite being unable to sleep. If this is the case, remain in the bed while doing relaxation exercises. If you are restless, however, or anxious about trying to sleep, or if you have a negative distraught association with the bed, the bedroom, and the ongoing struggle for sleep, you should get out of bed after about ten or fifteen minutes of being awake. Go to a spot outside of the bedroom. If this is not possible, go as far away from the bed in the bedroom as possible. This separation helps break the association of bed and sleep struggle.

Many insomniac kings used other bedrooms in their castles when they couldn't sleep in their own bed. Most of us, though, do not have this royal luxury. However, we often do have the possibility of the living room, or a chair or lounge in the bedroom or, if none of these are available, the bedroom floor.

Actually, many insomniacs seem to prefer the floor. The stretching out necessary to accommodate the hardness of the floor surface, plus the softness of rugs, seems to soothe and relax them. Some people favor the surface of a futon on the floor as an auxiliary bed when faced with a sleepless night. Many travelers report sleeping beautifully on these mattresses in Japan, whereas they are fitful sleepers or insomniacs at home.

When you get out of bed during cold weather it is wise to don a robe or carry a blanket with you to the other room. Otherwise, experiencing the shock of a low temperature may prove too arousing.

* * *

The spectrum of relaxation exercises, aside from those involving breathing, are divided into the following categories: physical techniques; relaxing imagery; counting and calculations; verbal relaxation exercises; visual relaxation exercises; and soporific sleep aids. All these relaxation techniques can be combined. The sleep seeker is advised to try a number of them, finding those exercises (or the combinations) that work best. It is important, however, not to become too obsessive and perfectionistic in using these procedures. Such zeal is likely to undo the relaxation attempts and, through performance anxiety, increase arousal. Try to be as cool and laid back as possible in doing these exercises.

You should not be an obsessive clock watcher at night. For an insomniac the sense of frustration with sleep loss can be intense and, to avoid this discombobulation, clocks should be turned to the wall. If an alarm clock is needed, put it under the bed to be heard, but not seen. To be sure of getting up on time rely on alarms. If you are afraid of oversleeping, use multiple alarm clocks or snooze alarms with repeated waking signals, or depend upon a wakeup phone service, sleep partner, or some other household member to awaken you.

Physical Relaxation Exercises

We begin with the physical methods. There are two kinds, the Day and the Jacobson techniques. In the Day method, muscles are relaxed progressively from the toes and the feet to the top of the head. While lying on your back in bed, or sitting comfortably in a chair, you should mentally will the muscles of the toes, feet, and ankles to unwind; wait until there is a loosening feeling in them and your feet seem to rest on the mattress or floor only under the influence of gravity, without muscle tension. When the feet have been relaxed, continue the loosening-up process with the lower legs, knees, and thighs, and then upward along the body. At each station and region of the body, try to will your muscles to relax and wait until you feel the heaviness of their loss of tension. While doing this, remember to continue to breathe slowly in and out through your nose. This exercise may be repeated three or four times until most of the musculature of the body is sufficiently untensed.

The second physical relaxation method is Jacobson's. In this method, a muscle group is contracted and the clenching in doing this is sustained until there is a mild amount of pain or strain; then the muscles are relaxed and a feeling of relief follows from loosening of the muscles. This exercise can be done using flexion at the ankle, knees, elbows, or neck; do the exercise twice at each location. Most people, however, prefer to do this exercise using only the making of fists, holding them clenched until they feel mild pain and then unclenching.

Some experts advise that physical relaxation exercises be continued for a number of weeks, night after night, until the ability to relax easily really takes hold. I have found physical relaxation methods to be of some help for insomniacs in their quest for sleep, but they are not entirely sufficient to achieve relaxation in all cases. They are most helpful in the case of individuals who experience a great deal of body tension in their sleep pursuit. I find that the following exercises are more immediately helpful for most people.

Use of Relaxing Imagery

First there is the use of relaxing imagery. Some people like to do their thinking in terms of pictures. Predominant are people who use this way of thinking in their work lives: artists, sculptors, photographers, and designers of many kinds. For this group, the use of the following images is suggested to help the relaxation process: Picture in your mind a leaf or a feather slowly falling to earth, being moved here and there by a gentle breeze and gradually drifting downward. The downward motion helps to lull you into the sleep state. Going upward opposes gravity and causes arousal. It is important in imagery exercises to focus on details, heightening the experience.

Another useful mental image is to picture oneself floating on a cloud or swinging gently in a hammock. Visualizing oneself in bucolic scenes with meadows, grass, and blue skies can also be tranquilizing. Resting in a cabin in front of a fireplace while the snow falls gently on the wooded forest outside is another soporific image. Or think of yourself relaxing on the beach, hearing the waves, breathing the salt-laden air, and watching gulls weave on a benign breeze. Similarly, sitting in a garden, seeing the flowers, smelling them, looking at green swards, and letting the sun warm you can be effectively somnolent for some. Those who like music that is soothing and conducive to unwinding may imagine themselves in an auditorium in a comfortable seat with the lights lowered, listening to a string quartet or an ensemble playing soft mood music.

For those who wish to combine imagery with physical relaxation, an effective tactic can be to do bodily relaxation at the same time that one visualizes colors. For example, you can relax the feet, while visualizing the color purple. Or try to relax the thighs to the mental image of the color nile green.

Visual Exercises

There are other recommended exercises for the visual thinker. Imagine a small black ball the size of a handball beginning to roll slowly toward you from the far distance, gradually increasing in size, until it is taller than you as it comes near you. A classic exercise is counting sheep jumping over a stile. You can also imagine yourself beside a railroad track as trains pass, counting the cars as they go by from the west to the east; then reverse directions and count the cars moving from the east to the west. Or imagine yourself descending a flight of stairs counting as you go down, starting on the top with step ten and then going to step nine, step eight, step seven, etc. Again, this exercise utilizes the sleep inducing gradient of descent.

For the visually oriented person another good technique is to imagine that you are standing before a blackboard with chalk in your hand. Then, mentally, draw a large circle about three feet in diameter on the board. If you are right-handed, draw the circle in a counter-clockwise direction; if you are left-handed, do it clockwise. The idea behind this exercise is to induce some sense of strain. Write the number 100 in the circle and then, using an imaginary eraser held in the opposite hand, erase the number while saying "I am sleepy." Then write the number 99 in the circle. Repeat the procedure from 100 on down, continuing as long as necessary until you are asleep. A related exercise is to draw a tic-tac-toe box on an imaginary blackboard and fill it in with x's and o's. Erase when all the boxes are filled in, and then start the game anew.

Calculations

Visual techniques work best for people who are facile with such imagery. Numerical exercises, on the other hand, are good for those who find doing calculations somewhat boring and therefore conducive to sleep. Start, for example, with the number 200 and slowly count down by ones as far as necessary until sleep intervenes. If this countdown is too short to work, start at 500 and repeat the process. A variation is "serial subtraction." Starting at 100 subtract 3 serially all the way down to 1 (100 -97, -94, -91, and so on).

Other calculation exercises can be invented and utilized by the creative sleep seeker, such as subtracting 9 from 100, then subtracting 8, then 7, and so on. Vary the tactic by subtracting 4, then 2, etc. All sorts of permutations and combinations on this simple but effective subtraction exercise can be tried out.

A more difficult arithmetic exercise is the following: From the figure 237, subtract 18 serially as far as possible. However, this exercise can be made easier by utilizing the following trick. Subtract 20 instead of 18; then add 2 to this result, thereby actually only subtracting 18. Continue to do this all the way down.

If your sleeping partner is sound sensitive, these exercises should be done only mentally. If the partner is a deep sleeper, you can do them in a low murmur, or even out loud if nothing seems able to arouse your bedmate.

These counting procedures are extremely successful as sleep inducers, yet in the hands of people with a tendency to be obsessive, they can lead to perfectionistic strivings; they should not be utilized if you find they cause arousal and further sleep difficulty. People who are good with numbers should not elaborate these exercises into complex, over-demanding tasks. They will then lose their boring and sleep producing effect.

Verbal Methods

Verbal methods can also be quite effective in producing sleep promoting relaxation. The simplest of these exercises are analogous to the counting methods in that they proceed in a serial way, and depend on monotony and boredom for their effect.

Imagine a nonsense syllable "AB." In front of this, mentally place the letters of the alphabet progressively from A to Z and pronounce each resulting nonsense syllable. For example, add A making this "AAB." Pronounce that. Then substitute B for the A. The resulting syllable is "BAB;" pronounce it. You can go through the alphabet all the way to "ZAB."

Another exercise is "alphabet repeat." It was taught to me by the ninety-eight-year-old insomniac whose sleep problem I've de-

scribed. His technique involved the recitation of the alphabet serially from A to Z, with the condition that all preceding letters
should be pronounced before saying a new one, concluding with
the letter itself, thus A, B(AB), C(ABC), D(ABCD), E(ABCDE),
F(ABCDEF), and so on.

The following exercises are wider in scope and less dependent
on serial progression. The first is to name the states of the U.S., by
letter, from A to W. There are no X, Y, or Z states. Visualize the
map of the U.S. and then locate the A states going from the Atlantic
Coast to the Midwest and then the West. Continue with each letter,
naming the states beginning with each letter and counting the total
accumulated at the same time, making sure that you wind up with
the sum of 50. Experts in geography can simultaneously name the
capitals of the individual states. Since the aim of these exercises is
boredom, it is not necessary to be perfect and to name each and
every state. A related geography exercise is to name the major
rivers, or waters (gulfs, seas, or oceans), of the world utilizing the
alphabet. Start with the letter A, naming the Amazon. The B river
is the Brahmaputra in India, C is the Congo, etc.

Another geography exercise involves visualizing a map of the
world and trying to name as many countries as you can. Begin
systematically with South America, going up to Central America,
the Caribbean Islands, Canada, Iceland, the Arctic, sweeping over
to Ireland, Great Britain, on to the European Continent, and thus
around the globe.

Another exercise involving the alphabet is to think of as many
feminine or masculine names as possible by the letter of the alphabet. Naming sports teams in a given league, including their
coaches, is a sports-oriented exercise. Any other individual area of
interest can be similarly used.

Sleep Aids

A group of relaxation techniques involves the use of sleep aids.
Many large book chains in the U.S. carry audio cassettes of a hypnotic nature that some people find helpful in attaining a relaxed
state. These tapes can be played on a tape recorder placed near
the bed; the recorder should be one that shuts itself off automatically, not requiring a possibly awakening movement on the part of
the listener. If sleeping with a bed partner who is sensitive to

sound, you can use the simple button hearing attachment that comes with many recorders and insert it lightly in the ear. When you fall asleep and turn in the night, this button falls easily out of the ear and out of the way, having accomplished its purpose.

Some people find it relaxing and sleep engendering to listen to all-night radio talk shows. For those not charmed by these marathons, relaxation tapes, music tapes, or general reading tapes may be of help, provided they are not too arousing.

Other practices that can help you relax are to read a book you couldn't seem to finish, play solitaire, or do crosswords. Physically, using small hand or body movements is soporific, as people who do small chores, needlepoint, ironing, and other tasks have found.

Insomniacs are often helped by doing puzzles or other boring or relaxing practices. These can be useful, up to a point. Sometimes, however, such activities become associated in the insomniac's mind with the difficulty of getting to sleep, just as the bed itself does. In these circumstances, it is important to change the pattern and do something different.

There are a host of other relaxation techniques and sleep aids available to people who have sleep problems. Biofeedback has been recommended for those exhibiting high muscular tension. Hypnosis, autohypnosis, acupuncture, are mentioned favorably by some. These and other techniques usually require special training or equipment, but, if available and desired, can be included in addition to the simpler, effective ones I have described.

Stress Reduction Techniques

Stress reduction techniques also are of service in the quest for relaxation and sleep induction and proceed on several fronts:

1. The environment—Escape or change a stressful situation, e.g., walk out of the room during an argument to decompress it.

2. Perception—Learn to think differently about stressful predicaments by eliminating irrational thinking, or thinking more positively, or acting more assertively in dealing with it.

3. Physiological reaction—Build up the body's resistance and readiness for dealing with stress through exercise, good hygiene (including sleep hygiene), and nutrition.

4. A further good practice is better time management by avoiding rush deadlines and scheduling more time for yourself. A list of

stress management dos and don'ts should include things like avoiding perfectionism, doing one thing at a time, knowing limits and when to say no, and tactfully venting feelings.

5. Identify sources of stress by their linkage with the physiological or mental reaction that indicates stress (sweaty palms, rapid heartbeat, anxiety, withdrawal). After identifying the source, behaviorist therapists recommend that you fill out a 3 x 5 file card with date and time and brief description of stress, nature of reaction symptoms, and statement of a plan to manage the stress situation. Cards should be completed before sleep time and action taken the next day. In other words, file and forget till dawn.

Chapter 10

Sleeping Pill Use and Misuse

For most of us, a pill is the concrete symbol of modern medical treatment. If we have pain, suffer from infections, need hormones or other substances which the body can no longer produce naturally, are afflicted by cardiac or ulcer complaints, or suffer anxiety or depression, we have recourse—usually successful—to medication in pill form, supplied by a physician.

If you are a sleep deprived person, however, you have no such winning resource. One-third of the population experiences sleep difficulties; and half of that number are motivated enough by their distress to take their problem to a physician. Half of this latter group receive prescriptions for sleeping pills. This statistic does not include the mass of over-the-counter preparations, street and recreational drugs, and alcoholic nightcaps that are turned to for sleep. Despite this demand, there is as yet no sleeping pill available which is totally without adverse effects on sleep physiology or other body functions, or which continues to work successfully for long periods of time. This does not mean that you cannot be helped by medication in the search for sleep. It merely means that a simple pill for solving your chronic insomnia is not yet available at your drugstore.

In the ancient and medieval worlds the search for substances that improved sleep (known as hypnotics) focused on plant remedies. To this day chamomile, valerian, and a host of other soporific herbs are relied on by many in their search for a good night's sleep. Today, the products of pharmacology and chemical technology are the most commonly used resources for sleep enhancement. Although a wide range of sleep promoting drugs is currently available, despite this plethora, difficulties remain. Problems of safety, negative side effects, upsetting effects on sleep stages, dependency and addiction tendencies, interactions with other drugs, limited duration of effectiveness, and rebound and withdrawal complications all hinder the successful employment of sleeping pills for chronic insomnia.

The Tolerance Problem

The primary dilemma of sleeping pills is the short-lived honeymoon. Most have only a briefly effective action of about two weeks. The buildup of resistance undoes the sleep benefits and insomnia reappears. This resistance to the drug is called "tolerance." Since the drug is a foreign substance, the body will oppose its action by attempting to undo its effects. Eventually, in the case of hypnotics (sleeping pills), when the tolerance defense wins out, the sleep improvement caused by the hypnotic is undone.

When hypnotics initially are tried in favorable circumstances, the medication works, the stress subsides, and the sleeping pills are discontinued. In unfavorable situations, though, the stress continues and hypnotic use is extended. In this event, the sleep induction of the drug wears off because of tolerance, and insomnia reappears. To cope with the return of the insomnia, drug dosage is increased or a new medication substituted. Again, with continued use and increased tolerance, the results are disappointing. It is in this situation of frustration that the danger of medication misuse and drug dependency occurs.

To overcome the failure of the drug to work, there is a renewed desperate attempt to both increase the dosage and prolong its use in the hopes of recapturing lost sleep. This mistake is fueled by the tantalizing few good nights of sleep that these dosage increases initially allow.

A depressing pattern of frantic, ineffective drug use interspersed with sporadic periods of relief, and an ongoing search for other more effective hypnotics, ensues. This occurs despite the fact that at therapeutic levels of the drug an increase of dosage is not followed by an increase in effect. The final outcome is a drug induced insomnia. Eventually, the buildup of tolerance resulting from an increased need to counteract the prolonged use of hypnotics can be so intense and its effects so arousing that it will bring on an insomnia. However, in the insomniac's mind his or her difficulties are still caused by the stubborn persistence of the insomnia, rather than by pill misuse and the sleep disruptive effects of tolerance. The impossible quest continues. (Other aspects of tolerance will be covered later when we discuss benzodiazepine hypnotics.)

Paul Fiddler, a successful accountant, suffered from chronic insomnia. In his history he stated that for sleep purposes he was taking four times the usual dosage of a tranquilizer on a nightly basis. He had originally commenced the use of the tranquilizer for sleep at the time of a business stress, and continued to take it after he tried an abrupt discontinuance that produced withdrawal symptoms. The sleep logs showed sleep onset and sleep maintenance difficulties; a diagnosis of drug induced insomnia was made and he was slowly weaned away from the medication. After the first week of withdrawal his sleep began to improve gradually, and by the end of the withdrawal period he was beginning to enjoy sleep again on a regular basis without drugs.

Secondary Conditioned Insomnia

In addition to development of drug induced insomnia there is an associated danger with drug misuse. When a stress has been successfully overcome and the insomnia linked to it relieved by use of sleeping pills, a new stress may occur. The shortsighted sleep loser returns to the "lesser evil" of pill use to counteract a renewed persistent insomnia. Through overreliance on sleeping pills and their resulting ineffectiveness, the danger of a secondary conditioned insomnia arises. The nightly prospect of facing the frustrating pill failure conditions the insomniac to arousal, and the self-fulfilling prophecy of loss of sleep.

Guidelines for Sleeping Pill Use

Hypnotics can be briefly used for dealing with sleep problems in transient and short term insomnias, under medical management, with the guiding principle of discontinuance as soon as possible.

Medication, though, should be used only if warranted by the health, safety, and well-being of the patient, or if the situation is sufficiently disturbing to the individual. If the pill works, the drug can be skipped after a few nights and only reused if the sleep distress returns and again seems too burdensome. Medication should be discontinued gradually to avoid withdrawal effects.

When indicated, it is important to introduce the use of sleep medication early in the course of transient and short term insomnias, to insure the prevention of chronic insomnia. When a more chronic insomnia develops, it may require more extensive hypnotic use, but could result in the possible danger of misuse.

In chronic insomnia, other tactics are practiced. Careful evaluation of the cause of the sleep problem is fundamental. If drugs are decided upon they are usually employed intermittently, with use limited to two to four times per week and, at most, twenty per month. Drug holidays, periods of time when medication is withdrawn and discontinued, generally are scheduled for about a week every month. Dosages are prescribed in minimal amounts and not increased without supervision. These measures are needed to prevent the buildup of tolerance and the development of drug induced insomnia, as well as a possibly unwise dependence on the medication on a continuing basis. Longer term hypnotic usage requires continuing, careful management, including periodic followups.

The use of drugs carries with it the introduction of powerful foreign forces, whose total effects might not, at the time of use, be known. Thus the nature of the clinical situation itself is always carefully considered. In the case of a pregnant or a nursing woman, for example, where drugs might have an adverse influence on the fetus, the child at the time of delivery, or the nursing infant, drug use is avoided.

The hazard of additive drug interactions is of particular significance with drug and alcohol abusers, where combining drugs is common. The danger of a cumulative effect from using hypnotics plus drugs of abuse, means that any person with a history of drug dependence should avoid the use of hypnotics.

It should also be borne in mind that drugs may have components such as dyes, which are capable of causing an allergic reaction that will interfere with sleep.

The Placebo Effect

There are important therapeutic considerations in the choice of a hypnotic. For example, there is the possibility of placebo effects.

A placebo is an inert chemical which achieves its results through suggestion. Such placebo effects take place in about twenty to forty percent of drug use. Placebo effects are caused by the expectations of the user rather than by the effectiveness of the drug.

Hypnotic Types

Antihistamines

Antihistamines usually have the side effect of strong sedation, which is the reason they are used as sleeping pills. They are usually the primary ingredient in over-the-counter sleeping medications. The main antihistamine that is used as a hypnotic, primarily because of its strong sedative effect, is diphenhydramine. It is the pharmacological component in such OTC (over-the-counter) hypnotics as Benadryl, Nytol, Sominex, and Excedrin and Tylenol PM preparations. Unisom, another OTC hypnotic, contains a different antihistamine.

Their sedative properties will not be sufficient, in customary dosages of these preparations, to deal with severe cases of insomnia. They are, therefore, frequently used in excess to achieve the necessary level of sedation to be effective. This can lead to a dangerous toxicity, as they are not safe in large dosages.

In addition, there are side effects with their use which can cause complicating problems: constipation, visual difficulties, dryness, and agitation. Their anticholinergic effects may create difficulties in men with prostatic enlargement, and in those individuals with a tendency to glaucoma. In addition, the strongly sedative effect of antihistamines may result in excessive daytime sleepiness and mental confusion.

The effects of antihistamines are exaggerated by alcohol and other drugs. They are effective only for a short time in producing sleep and therefore not useful for middle insomnia, as their action peaks in one hour. Tolerance occurs with one week of use. The limited period of sleep, if achieved, is followed in a few days by wakefulness and a rebound of insomnia because of rapidity of the appearance of tolerance when antihistamines are used. Nightmares can occur, caused by a rebound release of dammed-up REM dream pressure.

When used properly, antihistamines may be of limited aid in

some insomnias, as in those occurring with addictions, or when there is itching or allergy that causes insomnia. But the possible serious consequences of thoughtlessly increasing the weak normal dosage to threatening levels, when the low dosage proves ineffective, is always a serious possibility when antihistamines are used as a hypnotic.

It should be noted that although the occasional and limited use of over-the-counter nonprescription antihistamines for sleep promotion may not be harmful, their continuing or excessive use as hypnotics should not be undertaken unless it is under the management of a medical practitioner.

Chloral Hydrate

A prescription drug often used for sleep promotion is chloral hydrate. This is an alcohol product, with a very simple chemical structure, that has been available for the last century. Chloral hydrate works in about a half hour and its effectiveness against insomnia lasts for a few weeks with continuous use before tolerance comes to the fore. It does not affect sleep stages. Its main claim to fame is its use as a "knockout" drug when combined with alcohol. Because of its safety in lower dosages, it can be used for the medically ill and the elderly if there are no medical reasons against using it, such as the presence of breathing problems. Dosage level in the elderly should be drastically reduced, since the effects of delayed metabolism of sleeping medication in this population can lead to a critical level of the drug.

The drug does not depress the nervous system in low amounts. It is useful for difficulties in falling asleep because of its rapid onset of action. Its unpredictability is a negative feature. In some individuals it works quite well, but in others it has no effect whatsoever. Skin rash and gastric irritation are other negatives. As in the chemically related ethyl alcohol, addiction is a frequent problem with continued use. The major danger is that it can prove lethal in relatively small higher dosages. Chloral hydrate is lethal at ten times the sleep dosage level, but deaths have been reported at only four times this amount. Therefore, it must only be used under stringent medical control.

Abrupt withdrawal can cause overwhelming nightmares.

Barbiturates

Prior to the recent introduction of benzodiazepine hypnotics (see below), the prescription drugs mainly in use as hypnotics were the barbiturates. The reason for their application as sleeping medication was their strong sedative action.

Barbiturates have short spans (three to seven days) before tolerance appears, are quite lethal in overdose, have long sedation effects, have high REM supression effects, and can become addictive. For these reasons the use of barbituratese has largely been supplanted by the benzodiazepines.

Benzodiazepine Hypnotics

The major hypnotics currently in use are the prescription drugs known as the benzodiazepines (BDZs). The BDZs are prescription drugs and were first introduced as tranquilizers in 1961 with such well known examples as Valium and Librium. Soon after their sedative properties became known, drug manufacturers began a search for chemical variations of the basic BDZ molecule to meet the unrequited demand for better sleep medication, and eventually developed a number of benzodiazepine compounds (Restoril and Dalmane are examples) with strong sleep producing qualities, i.e., hypnotics.

The current predominant use of BDZs as sleeping pills is due to their safety, their relatively few side effects, and their effectiveness. These qualities are so significant that they have, as a class, replaced most other drugs previously used for insomnia. Their chief negative side effects as sleeping pills are: residual sedation the next day, especially with long lasting types and, to some extent, with intermediate ones; amnesia; and the recurring anxiety, confusion, and insomnia in the varieties that have a short duration of action. Although they have a limited inhibiting effect on dreaming sleep, they strongly suppress deep NREM sleep. This effect makes them useful in treating parasomnias (like sleepwalking) which occur during deep NREM sleep. There are other significant negative effects associated with their use, including a limited duration of effectiveness, lowering of the general energy level, as well as diminished libido and sexual performance in some cases. There is also a mild tendency to intensify a depression, if present. All these effects are dose related, with higher dosages causing greater problems.

The Three Classes of BDZ Sleeping Pills

There are three major types of benzodiazepines which are used as hypnotic drugs: the short acting; those with intermediate action; and the long acting.

The duration of action of a drug is dependent on what is called its "half-life." This is defined as the time it takes to get rid of half of the drug present in the body. This can vary from three to one hundred hours for BDZs. When a drug has a half-life greater than six hours and this drug is taken daily, accumulation in the body will occur.

The short acting benzodiazepine hypnotic (Halcion) is active for only a few hours, generally four to six, because it is rapidly metabolized and does not accumulate. As a rule, this rapidity of metabolism means that short acting hypnotics do not have hangover consequences for mood, performance, or thought process the next day, and are used when there is a need to be efficient and alert at that time.

The major intermediate benzodiazepine hypnotic (Restoril) has a slow absorption and, taken at bedtime, needs about two hours to reach peak effect. It functions as a sleeping pill that is mainly beneficial for middle insomnia problems because of this two hour lag. When the insomniac unluckily suffers from a sleep onset and a middle insomnia concurrently, this intermediate acting BDZ should be taken at least an hour or two before bedtime. Since it takes two hours to reach peak effect, taking it at this earlier time will make it work by bedtime, overcoming the sleep onset difficulty; its continuing later action will simultaneously overcome the middle insomnia.

In some intermediate BDZs (e.g., Restoril, ProSom), their effects can even last through the following day. Memory effects and recurring insomnia potential are slight with an intermediate BDZ.

Long acting benzodiazepines (Dalmane, Doral) can have hypnotic actions whose effects can last up to three to four days. In fact, they work better as hypnotics on the second or third day because of the buildup of sedative intermediate metabolic products. This allows insomniacs to forgo pills on the second or third night and builds up their confidence in being able to sleep without nightly pill taking.

Next day hangover symptoms, including drowsiness, are commonly associated with the use of long acting BDZs because of their protracted effects. For those patients that have high anxiety levels during the day, this action can be beneficial since its sedative effect helps to reduce their daytime level of arousal as well as induce sleep. This daytime sedation, however, can be dangerous for those individuals who require alertness. In an automobile driving test over a weaving and narrow course, those drivers using BDZs hit the sides more often than those on a placebo. Therefore, short acting hypnotics are called for when full control of senses and a quick reaction time are required. Most users report they are able to adjust to the hangover effects of intermediate and long acting BDZ types, becoming less bothered by them as time passes.

BZD hypnotics show other characteristics that correlate with their duration of action. The usual period of effectiveness for short and intermediate acting drugs is about two weeks when taken every night. The long acting drugs remain potent for more extended periods with continuous administration before tolerance takes place.

Tolerance in BDZs

Tolerance develops rapidly in short acting types and somewhat less rapidly in the intermediate group. It develops much more slowly in the long acting types, taking up to four to seven weeks.

Tolerance effects cause two types of insomnia. In the first type, called Rebound Anxiety insomnia, there is a surging tidal–wave-like return of insomnia that is usually greater in degree than the original insomnia. The anxiety derives from withdrawal effects that arise when tolerance cancels out the sedative action of the hypnotic.

The second type of tolerance effect is called REM Rebound insomnia. When sleeping pills that have strong REM suppressing properties are used, dreams are suppressed. When tolerance undoes the drug, the previously suppressed dreams will surge back as nightmares.

The morning anxiety that sometimes follows the use of short acting BDZs results from rebound effects in the early morning, when the hypnotic wears off after only a few hours of action. In addition to anxiety, episodes of confusion and amnesia in the morning frequently occur. These negative effects usually last through the morning. They are unexpected, and cause consternation, especially when the drug has lasted long enough to grant a fairly good night's sleep. These effects may also happen with intermediate acting hypnotics but are not typical of the long acting group unless the latter have been taken in quite high dosages and for long periods. The pill taker should be aware of all such side effects in the use of short acting BDZs; and of the hangover detriments on daytime performance that accompany the usage of intermediate and longer acting types. In some BDZs with rapid absorption rates, an unpleasant "buzz," dizziness, and paradoxial agitation may be a product of the rapid action of the drug.

Memory Disturbance with BDZs

The amnesic effect was shown by a female patient whom I interviewed the morning following her use of a short acting BDZ sleeping pill. In the session we discussed her experience of morning-after memory problems following usage of the drug. She graphically illustrated the memory effect by leaving her briefcase behind in my office at the end of the session. I had to call her later and remind her of the lapse.

The memory disturbance with BDZ use appears not to be caused by the loss of short term memory—that is, the ability to recall immediately what has just occurred—but rather by the failure of memory consolidation. The failure of consolidation prevents the integration of the experienced material within the long term memory bank. When memory consolidation fails, the brain behaves like Teflon; nothing sticks.

Memory difficulties are part of insomnia itself. Fifty-nine percent of chronic insomniacs have memory problems and if the insomnia is treated, memory complaints diminish. In milder cases, some patients who experience these memory problems have an eerie ability to go about their business for a number of hours into the morning. They function well until the amnesic effects disappear; then they have the problem of recalling what happened to them in the three or four previous hours of the morning.

Antidepressants as Hypnotics

Some of the many drugs that are used to combat depressions have sedative side effects. In addition, most antidepressants have a reduced capacity for the development of tolerance. For these reasons they are frequently employed when there is need for a long term hypnotic. There are drawbacks to their use, like diminished sex drive and sexual performance. They cause side effects like dryness, constipation, and—in the senior population—an increased propensity for urinary problems and leg movements that disturb sleep. The major dangers associated with their use, although they are not too frequent, are priapism (lasting painful erections) and cardiac side effects. Antidepressants are also potent suppressors of the REM phase of sleep.

Cautions on Drug Use

It is, of course, necessary for drug treatment of insomnia to be under medical management. It is strongly recommended that if you are taking any sleep medications, you should be aware of all their actions, interactions with other drugs, as well as their side effects. You should read up on the medication when possible, as well as being careful to note the informational insert accompanying most prescribed medications. Your pharmacist or physician can be called if in doubt. Bookstores have volumes available which are written for the layman and describe the actions, interactions with other drugs, side effects, and the dangers of most drugs. I checked my local bookstore recently and found three books of this type.

The use of any drug is a serious business. Even supposedly benign drugs which have been in widespread use can sometimes have unexpected harmful effects. This has been seen in the case of phenobarbital therapy for childhood epilepsies, which was supposed to be harmless until recently, when it turned out to have unexpected negative actions. The recent experience with L-Tryptophan, a supposedly harmless amino acid that was used as a hypnotic and was found to be associated with the development of a dangerous illness and therefore taken off the market, is another case in point.

Avoiding the aid of sleeping medication if this treatment modality is prescribed by a treating professional can be considered to be a misuse. Too often a rigid inhibition against any drug use whatever has been inculcated into people, with the result that it makes many sleep sufferers jittery about such help, even when it is properly recommended. As a consequence, the possibility of a perfectly rational treatment that might help an insomniac to find a safe, easy way to solve a sleep problem is rejected. The basis for this prejudice is the assumption that the use of hypnotics will inevitably lead to dependence. Statistics on hypnotic use refute this assumption. Seventy-five percent of hypnotic users take them for less than two weeks. Sixty-five percent of sleeping pill users, in one study, took fewer than thirty pills in the entire year. Only a small number (eleven percent of pill users) take them every night. A recent finding is that unnecessary suffering and stress can lead to impairment of the body's disease fighting capacity by causing weakening of the immune system.

It is also important to realize that despite the widespread use of benzodiazepines for sleep, the incidence of abuse of these substances for their euphoriant properties is not very great. Dependence on these drugs may occur on occasion but, in insomnia, the BDZs are used primarily for the purpose of securing sleep and not to get high.

It is emphasized that the prescription drugs discussed and described in this volume should only be taken on the advice of, and in consultation with, a qualified medical practitioner.

Drug Withdrawal

The common withdrawal effects of BDZs are anxiety, insomnia, and restlessness, but these symptoms are most often minimal and limited. There are other possible consequences of withdrawal, like irritability and agitation. The intensity of withdrawal effects is linked directly to the rapidity with which the drug is eliminated. When a BDZ has not accumulated, it is able to be rapidly dispatched from the arena of action almost at once.

For most short and intermediate acting BDZs, withdrawal effects last, in the main, for only a few days, continuing thereafter in a declining muted way for weeks. If the longer acting BDZs cause withdrawal effects, it takes a greater span of time for these effects to come to the fore, commencing, finally, about two weeks after the drug is discontinued.

Withdrawal Techniques

When it is necessary to terminate a hypnotic that has been taken for some time, the recommended process is an extended one. It should take at least two to three weeks of gradual weaning from the drug to avoid withdrawal effects that are too disturbing.

The techniques for relatively painless withdrawal from a drug are based on gradual reduction of the nightly dosage until the drug is washed out of the body. The usual formula is fifty percent reduction the first week, twenty-five percent the second week, and twenty-five percent the following week.

Some people find that withdrawing cold turkey works best for them. They prefer the discomfort of the three to five days of fairly intense withdrawal symptoms—irritability, insomnia, headaches, flu-like symptoms and, in rare cases, seizures—to the lingering process of a tapered withdrawal.

Other techniques of withdrawal involve temporary substitution of longer acting types for short acting hypnotics. This acts by diminishing withdrawal effects through the replacement of the short acting drug by the longer acting one with its less intense withdrawal picture. The longer acting drug is then withdrawn later with relatively little pain. In some cases, use of drugs that diminish nervous system arousal are prescribed during withdrawal to muffle withdrawal symptoms. All these techniques should, of course, be employed under medical supervision. When multiple types of sleeping pills are used concurrently, withdrawal of each, one at a time, is the choice. Where sleeping pill use has been excessive, the process of withdrawal can be difficult. Turning to a structured professional drug withdrawal program is advisable in this event.

I have found that the most common problem in withdrawal from hypnotics is the following. When a withdrawal schedule is undertaken, the occurrence of withdrawal symptoms may, although lasting only a short period of time in most cases, be experienced as unendurable by the insomnia sufferer. Even though the sufferer may have gained only a few hours of sleep with the help of the sleeping pills, and even though these pills may now be the cause of the sleeplessness, insomnia sufferers are so sensitized to the fear of loss of sleep that they will, in very many cases, simply return to the use of the hypnotics after a short period of withdrawal. In their minds taking pills is a lesser evil than the upsets and discomforts of withdrawal or loss of a short period of sleep before the promised return of good sleep. They have become skeptics because of the failures they might have had in prior attempts to overcome their insomnia and have, as a result, limited reserves of patience.

They have to learn that the withdrawal process needs time and fortitude. The persons who elect to withdraw should be educated to understand that a relatively short period of difficulty can be followed by surcease from their symptoms. Since they already have been suffering from the insomnia for some time, the short period required by withdrawal should be viewed from this wider perspective.

The search for more effective and safer hypnotics goes on. In Europe, sleep inducing peptides, which are combinations of amino acids, are being utilized.

Another natural compound that is being investigated as a possible hypnotic is the hormone Melatonin, produced in the pineal gland located at the frontal base of the brain. This hormone is produced during sleep and is inhibited in its manufacture by light. It is currently receiving intense attention as a new possible nondrug sleeping agent.

New types of BDZs, antihistamines, antidepressants, and a number of other drug types are all currently under development to answer the call of the chronically sleepless. And new varieties, such as the recently introduced short acting non-BDZ hypnotic Ambien—with greater hypnotic specificity, effectiveness, and fewer negative complications—are always appearing at pharmacies.

* * *

We have discussed the major insomnia patterns, how to discover their causes, and ways to treat them. In the following chapters we will be dealing with problems that are involved in the important areas of The Sleep Disorders, Circadian Rhythm Disorders, and the special sleep difficulties of the child, adolescent, and older age populations.

Chapter 11

Internal and External Clocks

Jet Lag, Shift Work, and Other Timing Problems

What if you can't stick to the rules? Suppose you travel a great deal? Or perhaps you have a predisposition to be an "owl;" you prefer to stay up late and sleep late but must adapt to an early rising "lark" job? What if you are a shift worker, expected to be at your most alert when the rest of the world is sleeping? What happens if you are suddenly called upon to work an entirely different schedule? What can you do to deal with the inevitable disruptions of sleep patterns?

Jet Lag Effects

Let's begin with jet lag, that all too commonly experienced product of the age of 747s and the Concorde. Jet lag usually results in transient insomnia of only a few days' duration. The disturbance of the sleep–wake rhythm abates in a gradual and fairly normal way. Yet for busy executives, athletes, musicians, entertainers, journalists, and politicians who have to contend with frequent flying, the body rhythm disorganizations caused by their jetting around the country or the world may become serious enough to bring on a chronic insomnia.

Jet travel often involves several changes of time, forward and backward. For Easterners the most usual time zone changes occur flying to the West Coast or to Europe. To take the worst case first, if we leave New York at 7 P.M. the usual six-hour transatlantic flight puts us down in London or Paris at 1 A.M. New York time. In terms of our New York biological rhythm, we have just fallen asleep and are looking forward to approximately another six hours of sleep. In European time it is now 7 A.M., the sun has just risen and, for people there, it is time to be up, preparing for the full day's work ahead. By 1 P.M. London or Paris time the New Yorker, who up to that point would have been groggy and nodding out, at last begins to biologically awaken and prepare for a day's activity. But that night at eleven P.M. local time, when Parisians or Londoners will be ready for sleep, the New Yorker will still be up and on the go biologically, unable to enter slumberland.

If a New Yorker flies westward, arrival at a West Coast airport will be in approximately five hours. It is three hours earlier on the West Coast than it is in New York and the traveler arriving at San Francisco will have to go to bed three hours later than the setting of his New York biological sleep schedule, in accord with west coast time. In chronobiology language, this means a "phase delay" of the biological clock of three hours. (The eastward European flight entailed a "phase advance" of six hours.)

It is easier to phase delay than to phase advance because when we phase advance, trying to get to bed earlier, we are pushing uphill since we are not yet tired enough to sleep. In phase delay we have the advantage of being more tired by the new sleep time. Demonstrating this is the fact that it takes a period of about an hour and a half per day, per time zone change, to adjust after flying eastward (phase advance) and only one hour per day after traveling westward (phase delay).

The symptoms of jet lag are sleepiness, irritability, poor performance, and digestive difficulties. Headaches, difficulty in psychomotor coordination, and malaise are also common. In-flight factors such as reduced oxygen, excessive vibration, noise, and uncomfortable sitting and sleeping arrangements all make matters worse. Luckily, the effects of this latter group of problems clear up more easily than does circadian distress, usually being overcome within a day or so. Jet lag may have particular impact on the traveler over fifty. At this age sleep quality normally begins to diminish, making older passengers more susceptible to jet lag and other deleterious effects of flight.

There are a number of techniques for dealing with jet lag. The general principle is to accustom the body as rapidly as possible to the time framework of the new environment. On eastward flights to Europe from the U.S., for example, the traveler can gradually advance sleep time one hour each night before the flight date and eat meals, if possible, on the new schedule. On arriving in Europe, go to bed immediately, sleep for only two hours, have a day's activity, and try to be exposed to bright morning sunlight, which is arousing and, in application of the principles of light therapy, aids in advancing the internal clock. An hour's walk will provide a good enough dose of sunshine to help chase away the jet lag blues. Go to bed at the local bedtime that evening. If absolutely necessary, a rapid acting sleeping pill could be prescribed for the first night or two if you will remain in the new zone for five days or less. If remaining longer, it is better to allow natural adaptation to occur.

A number of other tips to deal with jet lag have been advanced. They are:

1. Allow plenty of time in the new setting for rest and adjustment.

2. In flying westward, exposure to late afternoon or evening bright light helps you delay body rhythms and enables later bedtimes. If flying eastward, bright light exposure should be in the morning (phase advance).

3. Avoid overeating and drinking alcohol before the flight. On board the plane, avoid alcohol—which is dehydrating—and drink plenty of water or noncarbonated juices. Dehydration inhibits body rhythm adjustments. Carbonation may cause gastric distress.

4. On arrival, schedule necessary work or touring activities at times when you would be most awake and alert according to at-home body rhythm patterns.

5. Exercise lightly on the plane by walking in the aisles, when possible, to overcome fatigue and the effects of cramped quarters. Dress in light, nonconstrictive clothing.

6. A jet lag diet has been proposed but not yet validated by all researchers.

Delayed Sleep Phase Syndrome

A different kind of circadian out-of-phase problem was presented to me by a university professor who called in a panic toward the end of August. He had a lifelong tendency to be a night owl and in his extended vacation period over the summer he had fallen into an atypical sleep schedule. He was going to bed progressively later than at the beginning of the summer. By the time he consulted me, he was going to bed as late as 4 or 5 A.M. every night and awakening around noon the following day. His panic arose when he suddenly perceived that within a week or two he would have to conform to the normal class schedule and be at his teaching post at 9 A.M. He tried desperately, in the short period available, to get to sleep at an earlier hour in preparation for the need to conform to the normal classroom time schedule, but his body clock, now set in a 4 A.M. to noon sleep schedule, stubbornly refused to accommodate this sudden demand.

During his consultation with me, I explained that the treatment for this type of condition would take one week, with the treatment consisting of going to bed three hours later each night, sleeping as long as he was now doing but being sure to use an alarm to awaken each day after that, and going to bed each night three hours later than the previous day. The three hours of phase delay adds to the ability to fall asleep easily at the new time each night. After a week his clock was reset to a normal everyday lights-out time, and he stayed on the newly established schedule from that point on. I went on my vacation at this stage and scheduled him for a followup visit.

When I returned I had a message from my answering service saying that he had called to cancel and that he was now sleeping on the new schedule, at normal times, going to bed at approximately 11 P.M. and sticking to the new routine that he had achieved after the one week's recycling. This technique is called "Chronotherapy" (time therapy). The rescheduling utilizes a sleep hour time delay of three hours later rather than earlier each day because, as explained, such a delay is less difficult than trying to go to bed when one is not yet sleepy. It was, of course, necessary, once proper timing had been achieved, for the professor to stay with the new schedule despite his owlish tendency to prolong the day and go to bed later.

The professor's problem represents a wake–sleep disorder called Delayed Sleep Phase Syndrome. Persons who are night owls are more comfortable and function better in the evening and nighttime than during the daytime. They get into the habit of going to bed later and later; they fall asleep easily and sleep a normal seven to eight hours before awakening late in the morning. Problems arise when they have to get up early to conform to a nine-to-five schedule.

Delayed sleep schedules usually originate early in life or during college. The tendency may be the consequence of an inborn difficulty in coping with the required daily need to reset the bioclock to a twenty-four hour period rather than continuing on its innate twenty-five hour schedule. Sometimes the owl problem is the cumulative result of parental overpermissiveness that allowed a poor sleep schedule, or develops as an unchecked drift to a late routine. In most cases the daily lag stops when the night owl gets to a three or 4 A.M. bedtime, at which point some degree of conformity with the requisite normal schedule is attempted.

Individuals with this syndrome sleep quite well if they can set their own schedule. If a night owl tries to conform with more normal morning schedules, while keeping to his or her own late lights-out time during the work week, the resulting sleep debt is made up by compensatory long sleep on weekends.

Intractable delayed sleep phase patterns can call for job or lifestyle changes. A more severe form of this syndrome exists in which the delayed phase drift cannot be controlled and stopped at three or 4 A.M. but goes on to a thirty-five to forty hour cycle.

Shift Work

The sleep phase timing difficulties of the shift worker are of a different nature than that of jet lag. The jet traveler adjusts to the time schedule of the common new environment. In contrast, the shift worker adjusts to a time schedule which is in opposition to the cues and demands of the common environment. Shift workers must sleep while the world is awake, and vice versa. Other difficulties in addition to insomnia and poor quality of sleep arise from this dislocation. Gastric problems are a major complaint of shift workers, created by stubborn gastrointestinal rhythms that cling to the old schedules and are not synchronized to digest food at the new meal times. Eight times as many shift workers run the risk of stomach ulcers and gastritis as do day workers. Night owls, with their ability to sleep well in the morning hours, have an easier time with shift work than do larks.

Another major complaint is family friction. Shift workers are at odds with schedules on the home front. There is interference with their role as a sex partner and provider of companionship and security. Because of limited contact with their children, normal parent–child interactions may be strained. Social relationships with friends and extended family become skewed. In general a feeling of social alienation comes with the territory. Women face double difficulties when they are required to maintain their roles of primary responsibility as parents, and managers of the home, and at the same time adjust to the handicap of a shift work schedule. Writers and artists who are night owls, as well as entertainers, restauranteurs, and performers, tend to fall into the shift work schedule.

Most shift workers, because of their tours of duty, get, on average, five to seven hours less sleep than they need during a typical week, attempting to make up this sleep debt by sleeping longer on weekends. They often try to maintain the normal nine-to-five schedule over the weekend. This sets up a timing pattern that leads to biological rhythm difficulties on Monday, when the shift work agenda is resumed. There is a tendency to make up for the sleep loss not only by the weekend adjustment, but also by napping during the day. More than fifty percent of shift workers nap at least once a week.

Shift work problems are accentuated when a sudden change in production schedules, for instance, means moving from a daytime work period to an evening or a night schedule. The greater and more rapid the change, the greater the degree of problems. Advancing age in shift workers also tends to aggravate sleep problems because of the greater propensity for sleep difficulties in this epoch.

Shift work problems are of major concern since about twenty percent of the U.S. population are engaged in vocations requiring shift schedules. Increasing recognition of the problems related to shift work has led to the attempt to modulate changes of shift in order to minimize the tendency for mood and work performance difficulties. Strategies that schedule workers in a "forward" direction by having them go to the evening shift, taking advantage of the natural tendency for phase delay, and then, if necessary, to the night shift, rather than to a more difficult and more sleep disruptive "earlier" shift, are utilized. Some companies give workers a week off between shift changes to allow them to readjust. If a worker goes from a day shift to a midnight to 8 A.M. shift, it takes about two weeks to readjust. During such a period of adjustment, he should make use of the technique I recommended to the night-owl university professor: Stay up three hours later each night. That strategy returned the professor to a normal schedule; for the shift worker, it will result in a better adjustment to an abnormal schedule.

Shift workers should also heed sleep hygiene principles. They should allow time for relaxation after shifts and before going to bed, follow the rules on caffeine consumption, and schedule meals at times that are compatible with the shift schedule. Setting aside specific times for activities with spouse and children will help head off marital and family friction.

Appropriately timed light therapy is of valuable use to shift workers who are having problems adjusting to a new work regimen. It has been found that wearing dark glasses when returning home in daytime after a nighttime shift, helps prevent the disruptive sleep advance effects of sunlight on a shift worker's idiosyncratic wake–sleep schedule.

Chapter 12

Major Sleep Disorders

The sleep disorders are a group of dysfunctions of an organic nature. They result from defects in the nervous system centers that regulate sleep, or from disturbances of other biological processes that are also intimately connected with sleep, such as breathing. This chapter deals with sleep disorders met with in clinical practice. The story of Dr. George Jacobson's experience that follows, will illustrate Sleep Apnea, a major sleep disorder.

Obstructive Sleep Apnea

Dr. Jacobson, a retired dentist in his late seventies, developed sleep onset and middle insomnia one year after vascular difficulties cost him the loss of vision in his left eye. Until then, he had always been a good sleeper. Of medium height and slender, he described himself as a very physical person, and had spent a lot of time playing tennis to keep himself fit. He was forced to give up this pleasurable activity because of his loss of vision.

He suffered from mild arthritis, and its pain awakened him two or three times a night. He was able to overcome this interruption to sleep by moving around. This seemed to reduce the pain and enabled him to fall back to sleep. He developed a more unshakable insomnia, however, by obsessing about his visual problem. The loss of sleep pressure from the lack of his customary tennis workouts contributed to his problems. A constant daily worry developed over whether he would be able to sleep at night.

His daytime schedule involved taking occasional half-hour afternoon naps. As a rule, he urinated once or twice during the night. In episodes of poor sleep, this increased to four bathroom visits.

He described himself as a restless sleeper. His wife told him that he jerked his legs at night. He stated that he found himself awakening at times during the night, snorting and gasping for air. Since his vigorous snoring disturbed her sleep, his wife had slept in a separate bedroom for many years.

Dr. Jacobson's symptoms are characteristic of many of the signs of mild to moderate Obstructive Sleep Apnea (a = without, pneu = breath). In apnea, breathing is interrupted by periodic blockage of the airway. This causes victims to choke periodically and leaves them gasping for breath. Although sleep apnea occurs in approximately twenty-five percent of men over sixty-two, this problem actually begins at thirty-five to forty. The symptoms are so light then that there are no complaints until much later in life.

Dr. Jacobson's case was mild. Its major effect was to cause an insomnia; he complained mainly about his many awakenings during the night. People with light symptoms stay awake longer after nighttime wakes than those with more severe symptoms. This occurs because they are not so chronically tired as the more affected victims. Later on in the course of the illness, apnea victims are so fatigued by the frequent breath stopping episodes that they can't stay awake long enough to remember the sleep disruptions.

The major complaint in the more severe forms is a profound daytime sleepiness. In serious sleep apnea, the ever present intense daytime sleepiness causes sufferers to fall asleep while traveling, in the doctor's waiting room, over the dining room table, sitting in front of the TV, at the movies, or listening to the stereo. A particularly dangerous situation is falling asleep while driving.

Another major symptom of sleep apnea is intense snoring. The snoring level can become so high that it will exceed sixty-five decibels. By way of comparison, sounds of seventy-five decibels and over can cause hearing disturbances. The raucous snoring shows a pattern of increasing rasping and volume, which then stops abruptly for a variable period that can range from ten seconds to two minutes. This period of silence is terminated by loud gasping snorts as the person struggles to recover breath. These episodes can occur more than thirty times per night, and even up to hundreds of times in a single night's span.

It was not only Dr. Jacobson's loud snoring that led his wife to press for separate bedrooms, but also his restless sleep. Apneic sleep is characterized by agitated movements and sweatiness. The sheets and bedclothing are usually disordered. Dr. Jacobson slept only in pajama tops in order to move more about easily at night. Persons with serious cases of apnea, unlike the average person, often fall out of bed. Thrashing about in attempting to catch their breath, apneics sometimes strike, and inadvertently injure, their bed partners. His wife was disturbed by occasional kicks from her husband's leg twitches when they were sleeping in the same bed, as well as by his snoring and restlessness.

Sleepwalking and -talking, and the assumption of odd sleep positions are frequent. He preferred to sleep on his back. This sleep position has negative implications in obstructive sleep apnea, as it favors the occurrence of apneic episodes.

Oddly enough, but certainly understandably, it is not the patient's complaints in the more serious forms that lead to professional consultation. It is the suffering sleep partner, exposed to the sound and fury of an advanced obstructive sleep apnea, who usually blows the whistle. For this reason the aggrieved, innocent partner must give clarifying testimony during the initial sleep consultation since the patient is unaware of his or her violent snoring, breath stopping, and restless movements at night; as well as playing down the patient's markedly diminished daytime alertness, morning headaches, and inefficient functioning. For those who do not have a bed- or home-sharing informant when an apnea is suspected, a tape recording during the sleep period will provide auditory evidence of the snoring, snorting, and breath stopping. Hypertension and irregular cardiac rhythms are critical complications in advanced stages of the illness.

The personality changes in severe sleep apnea include irritability, anxiety, and depression. These symptoms, as well as other mood and behavior problems, may interfere with a couple's relations. Diminished libido and sexual capacity, and occasional nighttime bedwetting, also contribute to disharmony.

Although most frequent at the senior level, apnea presents itself at other ages. It is thought to be an accessory, or important, factor in Sudden Infant Death Syndrome. Apnea occurs in children with enlarged tonsils and adenoids, causing sleepiness. Poor school performance, irritability, hyperactivity, and antisocial behavior are the predominant symptoms at that time.

Obstructive sleep apnea has many sources. A major one is mechanical; when sleeping on the back, the tongue falls against the rear wall of the throat. The subsequent blockage acts like a cork in a bottle neck, reducing, or even totally obliterating, the ability to take breaths. A similar obstruction of the throat occurs with enlargement of the soft palate or tonsillar arches. Swollen tonsils and adenoids can cause it in children. Fat deposits in the throat of an obese person result in narrowing, which accentuates the corking-up process. Narrowing also occurs with anatomical malformations and in allergic and infectious inflammations that give rise to swelling of the throat. In later years the strength of the throat may weaken and, during inspiration—like an aged building wall—there is a tendency for it to collapse. All these circumstances may combine or act singly to result in the symptoms of apneic choking and breath stoppage.

The fatigue of sleep deprivation and excessive nighttime restlessness adds to the number of episodes. Alcohol taken close to bedtime is quite dangerous, since it is a central nervous system depressant, increasing a tendency to breath stoppage. Therefore, alcohol and other sedative use is forbidden for those who have apnea. It should be borne in mind that sleeping pills, barbiturates, tranquilizers, and anticonvulsants have a similar effect and are dangerous when taken in conjunction with an existing apnea.

Treatments for obstructive sleep apnea include: losing weight to combat obesity; giving up smoking; change of a back sleeping position to the side; sleeping with the head and thorax elevated by using a hassock or raising the head of the bed; laser surgical removal of polyps, tonsils, and adenoids or an oversized soft palate and tonsillar arches, when present. A tracheostomy (creating an opening from the outside to the larynx to bypass the throat obstruction) is now rarely used except in very severe cases or in emergencies. The preferred treatment in major apnea is Continuous Positive Airway Pressure, a procedure whereby oxygen under pressure is provided by nasal mask to keep the throat passage open during the night. Splints to extend the jaw, and retracting devices to pull the tongue base away from the back of the throat, have sometimes been helpful. Warning devices that are activated when the sleeper lies on his or her back have also been developed and used. Insomnia, by itself, may be treated in uncomplicated apneics that have a sleep complaint.

Dr. Jacobson's insomnia was significantly reduced by attention to sleep hygiene principles. His difficulties in falling asleep were overcome by an effective utilization of verbal relaxation techniques. This success reassured him about his ability to sleep, reducing his sleep worries. Referral to a sleep laboratory affirmed the mild nature of his apnea, requiring no further intervention. This also served to reassure him.

Central Sleep Apnea and Mixed Apnea

Central sleep apnea, another major type of breathing-related sleep difficulty, is caused by neurophysiologic problems in the respiratory control centers of the nervous system. It manifests itself in a periodic loss of diaphragmatic and chest muscle movement, resulting in episodes of diminished breathing or even breath stoppages. The throat, though, remains open in central sleep apnea, unlike obstructive apnea.

Central sleep apnea does not cause excessive daytime sleepiness nor heavy napping. Middle insomnia with frequent nighttime awakenings is the primary complaint. The awakenings may be accompanied by shortness of breath. Central apneics are not overweight. It occurs equally in both men and women, whereas obstructive apnea is found predominantly in men. Snoring, if it is present, is not distinctive.

The use of a diaphragmatic pacemaker is often necessary in this condition. Tricyclic antidepressants, which strengthen the capacity of the lungs and breathing apparatus of the body to function, are also useful.

There is a third kind of apnea in which both central and obstructive types are mixed. Complaints in this form will be dependent upon the proportion of the different apneas present in the mixture.

Mixed types are frequent, but pure central apnea is reportedly a rare event.

Ondine's Curse

There have been many tales and myths dealing with the themes of sleep and breathing. The giant in Jack and the Beanstalk slept and snored in between shouting episodes. Sleeping Beauty is another example, as well as Rip Van Winkle and his protracted sleep reaction to alcohol. Dicken's Joe, the fat boy of The Pickwick Papers, is often described as an example of sleep apnea and, in fact, his characterization gave rise to the term Pickwickian to describe a special medical picture involving obesity and sleepiness.

One of the most engaging of all of these myths is the Ondine Legend. Ondine, a female water spirit, acquired a soul. She did this by marrying a mortal. But her human husband was unfaithful to her. In revenge, Ondine appeared as a water nymph, and kissed and clasped him so forcefully that he was unable to breathe, with the result that he died as though drowned.

This myth has been the source of many artistic creations, including operas, ballets, and prose works. The most well known is the play *Ondine, A Romantic Fantasy In Three Acts* by Jean Giraudoux. In medicine, Ondine's Curse is an eponym to describe an otherwise healthy patient who periodically loses the ability to breathe. This loss of automatic breathing is a result of damage to nervous system centers that control respiration. Ondine's Curse symptoms occur throughout the day and night, in contrast to obstructive sleep and central sleep apneas that happen only at night.

Narcolepsy

Narcolepsy (narce = numbing, lepsis = attack), a sleep disorder afflicting a quarter of a million Americans, with men and women being equally affected, is often first diagnosed in the senior population. Narcolepsy is not a disease of old age, *per se*, and actually begins in young adulthood. Its symptoms can be so masked in the earlier years, however, that it may not be definitively identified until well into later life. It often exists in tandem with sleep apnea, with both contributing to an excessive daytime sleepiness. It is unmasked when the apnea is successfully treated and the underlying symptoms of narcolepsy are exposed and become recognized.

The primary symptom of narcolepsy is an excessive, insistent daytime sleepiness accompanied by periodic attacks of falling asleep as well as episodes of muscle weakness. Many adults experience these symptoms but rationalize them away without being aware of the underlying cause. They often resort to consumption of large amounts of coffee and other stimulants to counteract their discomforts, never realizing that they actually suffer from a sleep disorder.

Narcolepsy, in addition to its frequent correlation with sleep apnea, is also associated with nocturnal myoclonus (leg jerking) in half of its cases.

Daytime symptoms predominate in narcolepsy. These symptoms are of four kinds:

1. *Sleep attacks* during the day, which last from one to fifteen minutes, after which the sleepers awake refreshed and rejuvenated for about an hour. These attacks are often accompanied by dreams. Narcoleptics are abnormally drowsy throughout the day with diminished alertness and poor job performance. Sleep attacks can occur while driving (known narcoleptics give up driving licenses), after heavy meals, during socialization and sex, and with boring sedentary activities.

2. *Cataplexy* (cata = down, plexis = strike) is the other major symptom of narcolepsy. Its usual manifestation is a loss of voluntary muscle tone for a few seconds, that causes sagging or falling. It is frequently triggered by sudden intense emotions including fear, surprise, anger, or laughter. Consciousness is not lost during cataplexy since the person remains awake.

3. *Sleep paralysis* occurs for periods of about thirty seconds to ten minutes. The afflicted, though awake, can't open their eyes or move their limbs, and breathe with difficulty. These attacks take place at times of falling asleep or waking, and are not causally correlated with emotions. When they first happen, they are anxiety-provoking and accompanied by a fear of dying. The episodes of paralysis end spontaneously, but may also be terminated by someone's touch, or by forced blinking. In sleep paralysis there is a feeling of being weighed down, and a frightening frustration at not being able to move.

4. *Hypnagogic hallucinations* (hypno = sleep, agogic = moving toward) are dreamlike states which take place in the interval between sleep and waking. Unusual visual and sensory experiences occur during the episode, which ends spontaneously, and rarely lasts longer than a few minutes. These phenomena can be quite terrifying. The visual images are usually simple forms, circles or triangles, that get larger or smaller. They may also be more complex, consisting of animals or persons. The images are often colored. There may be auditory hallucinations, which at times have a threatening quality. Or they may just consist of a collection of sounds, although even an organized melody may be heard. Some-

times there are "out of body" experiences, with feelings of looking down on the body or of floating. There is a general sense, in these events, of danger and threat which causes great fright, especially if accompanied by sleep paralysis, as often happens. Since closing the eyes can bring on these episodes, the fear of doing this may lead to sleep onset insomnia. Blinking to see light and normal surroundings is a tactic that is used to wipe out the advent of the frightening images. The term hypnopompic (hypno = sleep, pompic = usher out) hallucinations is applied when the attacks occur upon awakening.

Although the full-blown picture consists of all four elements, usually only the symptom of the loss of muscle tone of cataplexy accompanies the main complaint of daytime sleep attacks. The other symptom elements may occur singly or in varied combinations.

The cause of narcolepsy is unknown, but is presumed to be organic in nature. In narcolepsy, the REM phase is a "loose cannon," occurring out-of-phase as an intrusion during daylight hours. Disturbed nighttime sleep with middle or sleep onset insomnia—owing to restlessness, and lightness and fragmentation of sleep—is increasingly evident as the person grows older.

The distinctive feature of nighttime sleep, as well as the daytime sleep attacks, is that sleep atypically begins with an almost immediate REM episode, rather than with a typical NREM period.

Narcolepsy can be extremely debilitating. There are interpersonal difficulties, and social life is circumscribed. Psychologically, depression is often present because of life limitations. Since emotion can trigger an attack, the need to inhibit it results in a washout affect, and a resulting masklike facial appearance. Psychotherapy and good support networks are of great help to the narcoleptic.

Stimulants, as well as scheduled short periodic naps, help counter daytime sleep attacks, but stimulants may produce a poor night's sleep. Nonsedating antidepressants, which reduce REM, are used to deal with the other symptoms of narcolepsy. Both the antidepressants and the stimulants may lead to decreased libido.

A recent provocative finding is the presence of an immune antigen in narcoleptics—an additional marker affirming the presence of narcolepsy. The significance of this is being investigated.

The Multiple Sleep Latency Test (MSLT) detects and measures excessive daytime sleepiness, and is used to diagnose narcolepsy.

Polysomnography, the EEG monitoring of brain waves in sleep, is employed in this test. Beginning at about 11 A.M., after a good night's sleep, the patient lies down in a darkened room for four separate nap periods, each about twenty minutes, taking place at two hour intervals. These periods are recorded. The average time it takes to fall asleep in these test periods is calculated and compared with normal values for the test person's age. For adults, a figure of less than five minutes of sleep latency shows the presence of excessive sleepiness. The test also demonstrates that in narcolepsy, REM (rapid eye movement) begins within ten to fifteen minutes of falling asleep, whereas the normal time for this is an hour or longer. This early onset of REM does not occur in other sleep disorders that show excessive daytime sleepiness, like obstructive sleep apnea, and serves as a distinguishing diagnostic marker for narcolepsy.

Restless Legs

Restless legs is a term describing a cryptic phenomenon of unknown cause. It has been attributed to many sources, including excessive caffeine use, low iron levels in the blood, an unknown neurological origin, and a variety of other possible etiologies. It may crop up during the day when the individual is at rest, or on lying down at night prior to sleep.

There is a family incidence in seventy-five percent of the cases. The disorder is fairly common, and the condition makes its appearance in the adult years, with attacks occurring more frequently in later years. The onset of an attack usually accompanies inactivity such as occurs on long drives, sitting for an extended period, and in sleep. Women are afflicted more often than men because of a correlation with menses, pregnancy, and menopause. The reason for this connection is unknown. It usually is responsible for sleep onset insomnia, but middle insomnia is also fairly frequent. When restless legs occurs during sleep, it awakens its victim, causing the middle insomnia. Both insomnias are followed by excessive sleepiness the next day. Sufferers are known as "nightwalkers" since they are so aroused by their aching legs that they walk the floor night after night, an activity that tends to relieve the symptom.

Restless legs produces an unpleasant feeling in the lower limbs, that often has a tendency to spread and may even rise to involve the trunk and the arms. The nature of the feeling is difficult to pin down descriptively. It is an achy, expanding, unpleasant sensation which the sufferer, by experience, knows can be relieved by movement, thus giving rise to the name of restless legs. There is an urge to move around in bed, get out of bed, walk around, stomp and shake the legs, and even run in place to undo the unpleasant sensations. A woman with this disorder did the Charleston in her bedroom at night to shake the symptom away.

Lois Browne, a violinist who plays in a string quartet, suffered from restless legs. In her case, of course, her prolonged sitting during performances set off attacks that were sheer torture, since they could not be relieved by walking. Proper medication (low dose opiate), taken before performances, allowed her to play without any outbreaks of the symptoms.

I have found that temperature plays a role in this condition. Cold weather catalyzes the incidence of the phenomenon; warmth tends to counteract it. Patients report that lying on a surface with many hairlike extensions—such as velvet or corduroy or rough wool—seems to help, since the touch of their fibers may soothe and warm the distressed muscles of the legs. As in many complaints of unknown etiology, a variety of treatments have been noted to be helpful for this condition, including sedating medications such as tranquilizers and aspirin-type compounds. Sleep researchers have demonstrated that certain opiate receptors in the brain are involved in the restless legs phenomenon and that the use of opiates such as methadone and oxycodone (Percodan) and related pharmaceuticals are helpful in dealing with it.

The primary drug that has been found to be useful for treatment of restless legs is L-Dopa (an energizing neurotransmitter, prescribed in the treatment of Parkinsonism). In the few cases where pain is present in addition to the restlessness, Tegretol (commonly used to treat epilepsy) is beneficial.

Nocturnal Myoclonus

Nearly every case of restless legs is accompanied by repetitive leg twitches called Nocturnal Myoclonus (myo = muscle, clonus = spasm). Nocturnal myoclonus is now customarily referred to by sleep specialists as "Periodic Leg Movements in Sleep." In nocturnal myoclonus quick rhythmic movements of the leg take place, each lasting about half a second to five seconds, with such jerks recurring every twenty to forty seconds. This malady, with its idiosyncratic movements, is also called Jerky Leg Syndrome. The episodes of jerkiness occur in clusters, each lasting from several minutes to hours. There is extension of the big toe, flexion upward of the foot at the ankle and, sometimes, flexing at the knee and hip. The movement resembles a "hot foot" reaction. Episodes are more frequent in the first half of the night. They rarely happen in young individuals, but increase with age and are fairly common in the older age group. They may occur independently but, as noted, in most cases are correlated with restless legs.

Mild myoclonus may not result in sleep difficulties. In fact, fifty percent of cases have no complaints. But stronger and more frequent movements cause problems not only in the sleeper, but also for a sleep partner. As in the case of snoring, the jerking legs, as a rule, do not awaken the sleeper, although the problem may result in many brief but forgotten awakenings which cause an unrefreshing sleep. The attacks of jerkiness can be substantial, numbering in the hundreds during the course of a night.

Nocturnal myoclonus may be linked with sleep apnea, and can occur in muscle and nerve disorders and a variety of other medical conditions, like anemia, uremia, or rheumatoid arthritis. Tricyclic antidepressant use may occasionally induce it. Withdrawal from drugs has also been responsible for episodes of jerky legs.

Bed partners complain of being repeatedly kicked and awakened by the movements. In the morning the bed looks like a disaster area because of the agitated leg movements and restless night's sleep. Patients complain of excessive daytime sleepiness and poor nighttime sleep.

The periodic movements with their distinctive leg jerks help to distinguish nocturnal myoclonus (periodic leg jerks) from leg cramps. Nocturnal leg cramps are induced by contraction of the calf and foot muscles, the characteristic ballet dancer stance. They are relieved by upward flexing of the toes and feet, or by leaning forward against the wall with the feet flat. They do not have the periodic quality of nocturnal myoclonus, and episodes usually last longer than those in myoclonus.

A range of treatments have been recommended for nocturnal myoclonus extending from tranquilizers—that work by preventing awakenings—to opiates (Percodan et al.) and L-dopa, that reduce the movements themselves.

Chapter 13

Sleep Across the Ages

Childhood Sleep: Infants and Toddlers

The duration and pattern of nightly sleep is greatly affected by age. Children's sleep in the first weeks of life totals up to 18 hours a day, and is made up of many short periods throughout the day and night. By the age of two months, these periods are reduced to two to four naps over the day. At three months about seventy percent of babies are "settled" into a daytime wake and nighttime sleep pattern, sleeping through the night in one major stretch from night to dawn.

There are great variations in sleeptime needs in individual children, and some children may be extremely short sleepers with a built-in tendency to sleep less. This may sometimes cause anxiety in parents who think their child is not getting enough rest.

Despite individual differences in sleep needs, each child will be consistent in his or her sleep schedule from day to day. The most frequent sleep problems seen in this early period of infancy are caused by difficulties with settling.

Bodyrocking, headrolling, and headbanging usually occur in the first year but most episodes of these erratic presleep practices will vanish by age four.

Sleep difficulties in the second year are mainly caused by fears of going to sleep. These problems are linked to anxieties about separation and loss that come to a head in the second or third year, disappearing by the fourth. Napping time during the day decreases; by four or five most children give up the daytime nap and are sleeping eleven hours a day.

Parents may interfere in their child's development of healthy sleep routines when they are overanxious and do not set effective limits on sleep scheduling. If they are a quarrelsome couple or there is a problem with alcoholism, an unstable environment is created that will interfere with good sleep training for the child.

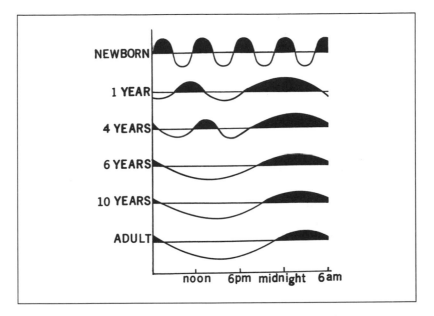

Daily Sleep Periods at Various Ages. By the age of six, sleep is consolidated into one session at night. After fifty there is a tendency (not shown in figure) for a return to a more frequent (polyphasic) sleep pattern. (Reprinted with permission from: Moorcroft, W.H. *Sleep, Dreaming, and Sleep Disorders,* Lanham M.D., University Press of America, 1989, p. 29.)

If the child is indulged too much by a little rocking or a little story too frequently granted at bedtime, this coddling can become a sleep onset association that bedevils a parent when the child awakens during the night and demands similar services at less convenient hours. If a contingency contract exists where food and drink orders are part of the deal, the effects of this gustatory reinforcement often lead to the little sybarite awakening four to five times a night, calling for refreshments.

Other disruptions to the child's development of good sleep habits can be environmental. Sharing rooms or beds with a child, or waking the little sleeper when arriving home late, are disruptive to good sleep training. The inevitable milestones of development that are met with in these years—weaning, toilet training, and starting school—may throw up road blocks to good sleep conditioning when they are linked to fears and anxieties that carry over into, and disturb, the sleep period.

The main danger signs that signal a developing sleep problem in young children are fatigue and irritability during the day, and the sudden loss of a previous ability to sleep well.

Middle Childhood

Many children develop parasomnias in early and middle childhood. These are out-of-phase events occurring during sleep that would normally take place during waking hours and result in partial arousal from sleep. They are usually the legacy of a developmental lag. They are phenomena of NREM, and occur in the first third of the night when the NREM state predominates. Sleepwalking, sleeptalking, and night terrors are examples. Bedwetting that persists beyond the age of five is also classified as a parasomnia. Tooth grinding, a frequent accompaniment of childhood, may last throughout adulthood, but most other parasomnias of children are outgrown spontaneously by adolescence.

Sleep problems in childhood are also often tied to environmentally caused difficulties (noise, cold, etc.), food intolerance (milk allergy), and pain. The pain of Sickle Cell Anemia crises are an example of the latter, awakening the child four to five times a night.

Neurological, asthmatic, and other respiratory disorders (including enlarged tonsils and adenoids that interfere with breathing), and middle-ear disease are other common medical problems that can cause sleep disruption in these years.

Delayed Sleep Phase Syndrome is a circadian rhythm problem that begins in early and middle childhood. It causes a slowdown of the child's biological clock. The braking effect can be a source of parent-child conflict when the parent—anxious about the child's compliance with school schedules—rushes the laggard little one in the morning. This time problem reaches a more raucous level in the next phase of development, adolescence.

Childhood-Onset Insomnia

A variant type of insomnia, called Childhood-Onset Insomnia, begins prior to puberty and persists throughout adult life. It shows a relatively steady pattern that has no correlation, causally, with intervening stressful events. Though its origins are unclear, it is thought by some to be the result of cumulative psychological difficulties. However, the consensus among sleep clinicians seems to be that it is connected with subtle central nervous system dysfunctioning. Childhood-onset insomnia is difficult to treat, although tricyclic antidepressants have been recommended.

Adolescent Sleep

The two primary sleep problems during the turbulent transitions of adolescence are difficulties awakening in the morning, and excessive daytime sleepiness. The need, at this age, to make room for an increase in social activities underlies these problems. To a degree, also, the biological clock slows down during adolescence. This circadian change results in a delay of sleep onset time and contributes to the tendency to sleep later in the morning.

The combination of circadian and life-style factors causes adolescents to stay up later and develop irregular sleep schedules. There is a tendency to oversleep on school days, and to have difficulty getting up for early classes. Usually adolescents come awake only at three in the afternoon. To adjust to the demands of their schoolwork under these pressures, they lop off sleep time, sleeping one or two hours less a day despite the need to make up their existing sleep deficit. And they frequently have part-time work after school, adding to their scheduling problems.

The sleepy adolescent attempts to compensate for the daily sleep deprivation by getting up late on weekends, but this can increase sleep hygiene deficits by adding irregularity to other disruptive timing problems.

Significant changes occur when students take their first uncertain steps out of the confines of a home environment and move to a college campus. The fixed home environment gives way to the transience of dormitory existence. Accompanying this new life are profound changes in the academic, emotional, and social areas.

These adjustments, and their stresses, are frequently reflected in an outbreak of insomnia.

A common sleep pattern is shown by the student who stays awake longer and goes to bed later. Lights-out time is delayed an average of two hours for the college student. The result is that many students have sleep onset insomnia when they attempt to meet early class schedules by going to bed at a normal hour.

The endemic reduction in total sleep time of the college adolescent tends to be made up by increased napping. The poor sleep habits developed in college can create problems when, after graduation, the new entrant into the work force must suddenly readjust to a rigid nine-to-five schedule.

Chronic sleepiness in adolescents is dangerous when they are behind the wheel, since most are new and relatively inexperienced drivers. This combination leads to the proliferation of automobile accidents that mark this period.

Since the activation of a delayed sleep phase syndrome is almost a normal fate for adolescents, many drift with the current into a pattern of using this tendency as an excuse for neurotic manipulation to have things their way. Students who want to miss school and don't really want to get up for classes will, for these reasons, turn off alarms and get belligerent if attempts are made to awaken them. These manipulators, who plead a waking problem, however, can easily get up by themselves on weekends if motivated by the prospect of a ski or fishing trip. They also show no problems with either sleep or waking during school vacations.

Adolescents experience sexual problems that may disturb their sleep. Guilt over masturbation, the effects of physical changes that are associated with puberty (like menses and secondary sexual development), and conflicts caused by sex temptations and problem-ridden sexual adjustments can influence adolescent sleep. The sometimes pernicious impact of peer pressure, the increased opportunities for smoking and alcohol abuse, and the cropping up of age-typical emotional illnesses—like bulimia or anorexia—are other problems in the passage through time that can negatively affect their sleep.

Those students who experiment with street drugs in their adolescent and early adult years sometimes develop disturbed sleep patterns when these drugs disrupt nighttime rest. To combat a resulting chronic insomnia "soft drugs" (minor tranquilizers et al.)

are resorted to, beginning a pernicious pattern of alternating street drug and hypnotic use. I have traced the origin of many persistent adult insomnias to this early abuse pattern.

Narcolepsy, a sleep disorder that begins in late adolescence and shows daytime sleepiness as its prime symptom, should be kept in mind when adolescents have trouble staying awake during the day. Drug abuse, laziness, or illness should not be the only possible causes to consider when there is evidence of excessive somnolence at this time.

Chapter 14

Senior Sleep

We reach the senior phase of our life cycle at fifty. The baby boom generation begins to cross this threshold at about the year 2000. At this time roughly 30 million Americans, approximately fifteen percent of the population, will be fifty or older. This age group numbered only twelve percent a decade ago. By the year 2020, the graying of the population is expected to increase to twenty percent.

Gray is not the only color we think of in connection with these advanced years, however. They are known as the "golden years." This is a time of wisdom, earned retirement from the struggle to win the daily bread, and the leisure to pursue knowledge, recreation, travel, and entertainment. An additional bounty is playing the role of family icon to the audience of one's descendants. However, along with these benefits increasing age also brings new stresses.

Sleep Changes With Age

It is estimated that five million older individuals in the U.S. have severe sleep problems, half of whom take sleeping pills from time to time, some of them on a daily basis. About thirty-five percent of the sleeping pills used in the U.S. are prescribed for this group. The figure is even greater for those in long term care facilities, where about ninety percent receive them nightly.

Diminished and less invigorating sleep is a normal physiologic part of aging, like diminished eyesight and hearing, wrinkling of the skin, and gray hair. About eighty percent of people begin to have shortened and lighter sleep at fifty. The eventual degree of sleep loss the senior population suffers can be substantial, ranging from twenty-five to fifty percent.

The predominant symptom that plagues the older population is sleepiness. The symptom is often the result of lighter, more broken sleep but is also attributed to abnormal breathing and leg movement problems.

The older population experiences an increase in episodes of wakefulness at night, with nighttime awakenings tripling by seventy. Sleep in the seventies and eighties is interrupted six to seven times more often than for those under forty, whereas the time spent awake at night increases, averaging fifty minutes in senior groups. An increase in the number of brief (fifteen second) wake episodes—which are too short to be remembered— reinforces the negative effects. These events are frequently associated with an increase in snoring and restlessness that cause an increase in partner complaints. The usual demoralizing insomniac feelings of helplessness, of subjective feelings of loneliness, and of being different than "normal good sleepers" accompany this increased wakefulness.

Older sleep deprived persons are much more likely to make up for lost sleep by daytime napping, but some cannot sleep at all during the day, even though awake most of the night. The potent influence of sleepiness makes itself felt in an increase in unplanned naps during the day; every period of inactivity, every instance of boredom, leads to spontaneous napping. However, excessive daytime sleepiness and the need for napping, even for multiple naps, may not be recognized as an indication of a possible underlying sleep problem by the senior insomniac.

The major villain responsible for diminished sleep among older persons is a significant decrease in stage 4, the deepest, most refreshing stage of sleep that totals 1.2 hours per night in the young adult but gradually diminishes to almost zero after the fifties.

In later life, the body rhythms involving sleep–wake cycles become less reliable and efficient and less capable of adapting. For example, body temperature, which is normally banked and at its lowest level in sleep, can advance in its rhythm and inappropriately flare up earlier during the night. An advance in sleep timing, a feature of aging, results in an earlier bedtime and an earlier waketime. This accounts for the older sleeper's tendency to awaken toward the end of the night, facing the dilemma of what to do in the darkness until daybreak arrives. Seniors, in general, are less tolerant of circadian changes and handle experiences asociated with them, such as jet lag, poorly.

Although retirement from the work force frees the retiree from the need to comply with a nine-to-five working schedule, this freedom can be a two-edged sword. The loss of familiar work schedules, social roles, and the reduced incomes that accompany retirement, engender fears of insecurity and the loss of independence. When no activities are found to replace the former structure and if healthy engaging group and individual interests are not established, there may be surrender to such passive pursuits as watching TV, napping, and a monotonous frittering away of the passage of time. The lack of activity and exercise under these circumstances, and the attempt to vary a boring existence by escape into napping, carry with them the danger of diminished sleep drive and its resulting sleeplessness.

The loss of spouses, family members, and friends and a threatening awareness and fear of death, as well as an increased amount of health problems and other upsetting physical changes, are further specters that haunt this otherwise auspicious period and can lead to sleep difficulties.

* * *

Mr. Gordon, a laborer, required surgical treatment of his carpal tunnel syndrome that affected both his hands. In this illness, thickening of the wrist tissue around the tendons that move the hands and fingers produces numbing of the fingers and limitation of hand movement. His operations were only partial successes. The physical difficulties that remained in spite of the surgery made it hard for him to obtain employment. He was forced to retire, and lived on a limited income. Although he looked hale and hearty, the loss of his ability to work was a severe blow to his role and image, and resulted in stress that eventually led to insomnia.

In another case Mrs. Singer, an eighty-year-old widow, found herself frequently awakening in distress at night, and fell into the habit of consuming a fairly large amount of food—which seemed to help her get back to sleep. She was moderately diabetic, but did not stick to the necessary diet schedule to control it. In addition she observed poor sleep hygiene by keeping irregular sleep hours, and was depressed by her illness and other aspects of her life.

Mrs. Singer's case illustrates a common psychiatric complication that is often seen in the later years of life—the presence of depression.

Her insomnia problem was brought on by a poor dietary regimen, which led to attacks of sweatiness (a symptom of low blood sugar, hypoglycemia) at night that awakened her. Her poor sleep hygiene and depression also contributed. Each of these causal elements had to be corrected, in turn, to undo her sleep difficulties.

* * *

The older sleeper is more sensitive to environmental stimuli like noise, lights, and activity, and is more easily startled out of sleep by them than is a younger person.

Nasal decongestants and stimulants (such as those used to control weight), caffeine (the effects of a cup of coffee may last over twelve hours in an older person) and some prescription drugs, are frequently implicated in sleep difficulties. Inappropriate chronic use of sleeping pills is a common problem, and the interaction of the increased number of drugs used for physical illness by seniors can have unsuspected sleep interfering effects. The attempt at self-medication to counteract daytime fatigue—by using caffeine, alcohol nightcaps, or a reflexive reach for pills to find sleep—should be discouraged.

Insomnia in women increases after menopause. In fact, in the later years women complain more than men about loss of sleep, with thirty-one percent of women in this group—versus only sixteen percent of men—describing subjective insomnia symptoms. Research has shown, paradoxically, that it is actually men who have an increased number of awakenings and other sleep disruptions.

Prostatic enlargement is a medical problem for most older men. Retention of urine, with heightened urgency and frequent trips to the bathroom, is a common complaint and an added impediment to sleep continuity. This problem is dealt with in many ways. Fluid restriction in the evening, use of drugs that inhibit the drive to void, the newly developed procedure of using hormones to shrink the prostate, and, if necessary, urological surgery are various tactics to deal with this common difficulty of the older male.

The ways in which seniors deal with sleep loss differ from those of younger persons. The latter are quicker to recognize correlations between their stress, anxiety, and depression, and their sleep difficulties. Older sleep sufferers fixate, instead, on their physical problems, like pain and fatigue, rather than on the role of emotional conflict. In fact, there is a tendency for them to deny any depression or anxiety. To an extent, this is primarily owing to the impact of the many medical and drug-related factors involved in the origin of senior sleep problems. There is a causal chain established in the senior life phase where illness and unfortunate life experiences lead to depression that secondarily result in poor sleep.

One must be careful not to chalk up the pessimism, insomnia, and body complaints of a senior person to "just growing old." Depressions in the senior group are very common, and should always be considered as a possibility when insomnia occurs in the later years. When seen in an older person the symptoms of insomnia, loss of appetite, loss of weight, loss of interest, fatigue, as well as associated negative feelings of hopelessness and worthlessness, are often signs that the presence of a depression must be taken into account and proper consultation with a professional is in order.

Depression in the elderly has a characteristically "empty" feel. Concerns about specific losses or traumatic separations, which are usually implicated in depression, are absent. Instead of concern about the underlying loss or trauma, the focus is on bodily complaints and insomnia.

Organic Neurological Changes

An oncoming age related Organic Brain Syndrome gives rise, in seniors, to difficulties in memory, rapid mood changes, periods of confusion, and sleep problems. These organic changes create increased wakefulness at night, and more sleep during the day. A special instance involves Alzheimer's Disease, where there is a notable increase in nighttime awakenings. In fact, laboratory sleep studies may help to diagnose Alzheimer's Disease in its early stages, being particularly helpful in differentiating it from depression.

"Sundowning" is a type of sleep disturbance which takes place in elderly people who are experiencing a mild to moderate degree of organic brain changes. In the sundowning individual, daytime functioning exists on a very low level because of diminished brain efficiency. With nighttime, a tendency toward disorientation, anxiety, and restlessness can occur. Sundowners wander around as though lost, trying to find their bearings. The absence of a clear, orienting perceptual structure results in an anxiety which ignites the sundowning syndrome. This may happen on awakening at night in a darkened room. The loss of familiar caretakers or well-known normal surroundings may be involved in setting off this nighttime wandering and agitation. There is speculation that sundowning may be linked to circadian changes, since it is associated with decreased daytime activity and with changes in sleep–wake rhythms. The upsets caused by nighttime wanderings, restlessness, and agitation can be an important family problem and a major reason for placement of sundowning seniors in nursing homes.

A night-light can be helpful for the sundowning person. If elderly persons move to a new bedroom, it should contain their familiar personal articles. Daytime activity should also be increased. The British system of "nightwatchers," with scheduled family members or hired personnel awake through the night and charged with keeping an eye on the sundowner, has been recommended to help deal with the problem.

A recent study of residents in a nursing home showed a correlation between diminished daylight and the amount of agitated behavior in the period from September to December, when daytime illumination drops. It was calculated that in September there was six times more daylight than in wintertime. Disruptive behavior was found to increase in winter, occurring mainly after sunset.

Irregular Schedules

The correlation of lack of work scheduling and the subsequent development of chaotic, irregular sleep–wake patterns, is frequently encountered in the aged. A number of factors are involved, including inactivity and napping during the day, frequent awakenings at night, the effects of sleeping pill misuse, and changes in wake–sleep and activity–rest patterns. The cumulative effect is fatigue that engenders a tendency to go to sleep earlier and awaken too early.

Irregular wake–sleep patterns, and related sleep schedule and insomnia problems, tend to perpetuate themselves. The irregularity causes an insomnia and the insomnia, in turn, adds to the irregularity. This dilemma is a common cause of the excessive sleeping pill use seen in the older age groups. Senior sleep sufferers frequently overlook or rationalize their indulgence in problematic, irregular sleep–wake schedules.

A study has shown that those with irregular schedules differ from the normal elderly in their behavior. Normals showed a transition from activity to a quiet, relaxed state at 10 P.M. The quiet state continued until about 8 A.M. the following day, at which point activities began again, rising steeply, to peak around noon. This high point was followed by a gradual decline in activity over the next ten hours with a marked dip occurring at about 4 P.M.

In contrast, older persons with irregular sleep–wake patterns showed significantly less activity during the day. Although their quiet phase also began at 10 P.M. it was not as smooth, and was marked by more sleep disruptive activity during the night. The low point for the quiet phase occurred much earlier, at 2 A.M., at which time sleep disruptive activity suddenly began with a sharp rise, which continued till noon the following day. The normal afternoon dip in activity was absent.

Treatment of Insomnia in the Senior Group

The solution to sleep problems in the older age group involves use of good sleep hygiene principles, with regular lights-out and wake-times.

Sleep hygiene programs should be adhered to for several weeks at least, in order to give them time to have effect. One nap during the day, preferably for at most forty-five minutes after lunch, is also in order for seniors. Since napping during the day adds to total daily sleep time, it should be reckoned in with nighttime sleep when estimating a total twenty-four hour sleep amount. Although there is some decrease, overall, in daily sleep with age, the total remains fairly close to that of younger ages if daytime naps are added to nighttime sleep. Multiple naps, as a rule, should be avoided. The older sleeper should be cognizant of the normalcy of the lightened and less refreshing quality of sleep that is typical after fifty.

Many seniors feel that the loss of their morning bounce is really owing to their inability to achieve an idealized eight hours of sleep. It helps them to know that trying to increase sleep by staying in bed longer and taking more frequent naps will make the problem worse, rather than better. The older person may sometimes revert to the early childhood pattern of having more than one daily extended sleep period. Keeping this in mind, it is wise to know that the primary goal for the older person is not an uninterrupted sleep, but better daytime functioning.

Activity and social events, paced to the individual's abilities, are recommended. Education and reassurance about normal sleep, greater participation in family, social, and community programs, plus the practice of good sleep habits are the first line of defense in resolving an insomnia problem in the advanced years.

Most sleeping pills prescribed for the elderly are given as part of the treatment of medical problems, where insomnia frequently occurs as part of the symptom picture. When hypnotics have been prescribed for an insomnia problem, they are given for short periods, in the lowest effective dosage. The elderly, though, often require long term hypnotic use.

Older persons have slower metabolism rates; drug use, in their case, may lead to increased perils (such as accumulation and overdosage). When sleeping pills are recommended for seniors, those having low levels of toxicity, lessened tendency to accumulate, as well as high general safety and minimum withdrawal effects, are the choice of prescribers. Special care that the use of hypnotics is necessary and not contraindicated is the rule for this population.

Short acting hypnotics (like the prescription drug Ambien) that remain in the body for only a few hours are usually written for seniors to prevent drug accumulation effects—like confusion. Drugs usually last longer in the elderly since they have a higher proportion of fat in relation to muscle, and hypnotics are stored in body fats. The increased amount of drugs used by seniors also increases the possibility of additive effects from the interaction of hypnotics with other drugs. Intermittent use is the accepted policy.

A drug holiday, with cessation of drug use following every few nights of good sleep, is the usual recommendation. Drugs that have minimal daytime hangover effects—such as interference with daily routine, and problems of uncoordination that can lead to the danger of falls and fractures—are usually employed. To counteract memory loss problems, a written drug schedule is useful to avoid taking extra dosages of prescribed medication. Drug tolerance is weakened in the elderly and this causes increased hangover effects.

All elderly patients taking hypnotics should be seen frequently and regularly by their treating professionals, especially when there is a change in medication schedule.

The use of antihistamines in over-the-counter sleeping medications should be avoided by the senior insomniac. At prescribed dosages they are relatively ineffective and there is the resulting danger of a temptation to increase the dosage which, as described in chapter 10, can lead to ominous effects. Seniors should also avoid the dangerous practice of using alcohol as a hypnotic.

Finally, there is a very common insomnia pattern in senior insomnia in which a period of good slumber at the beginning of the night is followed by a long sleepless middle period, followed, finally, by a return of sleep near morning that is often prolonged past normal waketime. "Sleep Restriction" is a behavioral technique that has been found to be quite effective in treating this type of insomnia. This technique is described in the Appendix.

Reports indicate that the use of light therapy in the late afternoon or early evening helps in the struggle of seniors who sleep in this pattern. This enables them to stay awake longer and helps them regain the ability to sleep throughout the night.

Activities that involve large body movements, like emptying out and rearranging drawers, or moderate exercise involving moving large body parts, are arousing and can help to maintain wakefulness and avoid an excessively early bedtime. Conversation, fresh air, and rousing music are also beneficial in staying alert and awake.

By far the most common insomnia pattern in the older age group is an early A.M. insomnia, mainly caused by a circadian advance in sleep timing. This form of insomnia is also seen in the depressions in seniors that follow the frequent medical illnesses and life stresses that come with aging. Gradual delay of bedtime at intervals of fifteen minutes a week, or light therapy in the early evening, or sleep restriction therapy, are ways to deal with this problem.

Chapter 15

Sleep Positions

The positions we take in our beds every night echo our ways of dealing with the daytime world. We sleep as we live. In an earlier book, *Sleep Positions—The Night Language of the Body*, I cataloged and spelled out the messages expressed by a wide range of individual and couple sleep positions. The unique patterns of personality which identify us in our work, social, and interpersonal lives as particular individuals, are also projected in our insomnia patterns.

I have found the knowledge of sleep positions and their meanings invaluable in the treatment of insomnia. Sleep position analysis provides helpful insights in the areas of diagnosis, etiology, and therapy. There have been many examples of the value of sleep position analysis in diagnosis and treatment interspersed throughout this book. The interpretations and insights derived from sleep position analysis expand the ability to overcome insomnia problems.

Tonight, discover your sleep position for yourself. Observe the position you spontaneously assume to make yourself feel most comfortable at the moment when you decide you are ready to fall asleep and enter the sleep world. This is your preferred sleep position. Knowing this position, and assuming it (in addition to whatever treatment program that is taking place), will help make the process of sleep recovery easier.

This chapter presents a brief review of sleep positions, as well as further clinical experiences that demonstrate the use I have made of them in my work in treating insomnia.

Sleep Positions Studies

Ancient Indian practitioners of yoga in the East left records of some representative sleep positions. In the early 1900s the sleep positions of Harvard undergraduates were studied. In the 1920s Alfred Adler and some of his psychoanalytic disciples also became interested in sleep positions, correlating some examples with personality types.

Sleepers were photographed in all-night sessions in research done at Carnegie Tech in the 1930s. Body positions were found to change twenty to forty times over the course of the night, each position being held for about fifteen minutes. The investigators were struck by the consistency of the positions, night after night, and the "unusual contortions" in which some subjects slept.

Since the publication of my book *Sleep Positions* in 1977, there have been many articles published on the applications of sleep position theory. The dozens of articles on sleep positions, and the wide range of applications in medicine, archeology, esthetics, literature, and forensic medicine are only some of the various directions this work has taken.

The observation that couples assume meaningful sleep positions naturally led me, in my book *LoveLives,* to the consideration of the meaning of sex positions. I found that, as in sleep positions, preferred sex positions reflect the individual personalities and the nature of the couple's relationship.

Contemporary Sleep Position Research

The premises underlying my interpretations of individual sleep positions have been validated by a recent experimental investigation. This study affirmed that sleep positions "may represent a basic shorthand to one's characterological structure and defenses and may be a valuable phenomenon to study for both its normal and clinical implications."

A Canadian research group, using all night time-lapse film recordings, followed up my work on sleep positions. Their studies established that poor sleepers changed positions more often and had more body movements during sleep than good sleepers, and that changes in sleep positions diminished with age. They also found an increase in the duration of positions as age progressed. The most frequent sleep position assumed by children was on the ack; the side position was most frequent in adults, while the prone position was chosen the least by all ages and was almost absent in the older age category. A later study by this group showed that insomniacs were veritable whirling dervishes, moving restlessly and often. Their agitated fretfulness was interpreted as an "unsuccessful search for a rewarding posture."

Several recent studies have been made of sleep positions in sleep apnea. This is an important issue since those who sleep in the royal position (on their backs) increase the severity and concomitant dangers of their apnea. Sleep researchers puzzle over the strong tendency of apneic sleepers to remain in this position, despite the breathing difficulties. A Chicago group attempted to decondition apneic royal sleepers by using alarms which went off if they remained on their backs for fifteen minutes or more, trying to induce them to move to a less vulnerable sleep position. A large number of these back sleepers, though, obstinately retain their position despite its detriment to their well-being, a testimony to the unyielding preference for a personal sleep position.

Recent statistical analysis and field interviews in Australia and in England have demonstrated that the prone sleep position, which had been recommended in the past, fostered the Sudden Infant Death Syndrome. On the basis of these studies they recommended a change, and suggested that infants be placed on their backs in their cribs. As a result of following this recommendation there was a marked drop in the incidence of sudden infant death where these guidelines were followed.

The Four Basic Individual Sleep Positions

In the Prone position the sleeper lies facedown with the arms extended, generally above the head. This sleep position is preferred by individuals who can be described as having strong compulsive tendencies in their personalities. Even in sleep, they must remain in hands-on control of their world, in this case the surface of the bed. They are precise, active, neat, somewhat rigid, perfectionistic, and scrupulous. They are careful in their actions, always seeking to maintain control of their behavior and their environment. They are doers, and tend to be early risers and short sleepers. They are quite successful in their lives and are generously rewarded by society for their activity and accomplishments. In personality they seem to be mainly compulsive and do well in professions like banking, accounting, business, and management.

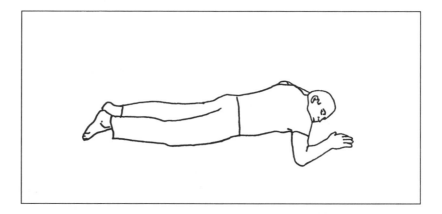

The Royal is the second basic position and is the polar opposite of the prone position. The royal sleeper prefers the supine posture, entirely upon the back, with arms somewhat akimbo at the sides. These sleepers are open and expansive in their personalities and display great self-confidence. An only child, or the youngest child, or the most favored child in a family often selects this sleep position. These children may be truly said to be the royalty of the family. Such sleepers display a high degree of self-involvement, healthy or otherwise, and could be said to have narcissistic tendencies. Whereas bankers, accountants, and administrators prefer the prone position, the royal position is more typical of actors, TV hosts, and other extroverts. It is called royal since it was also the position assumed by medieval kings when giving audience to their subjects.

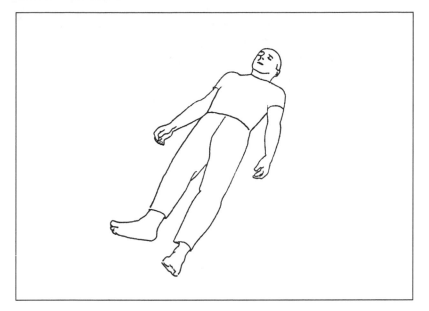

The third basic position is the Semi-Fetal, the most common one of all. These sleepers lie on their sides with knees slightly bent. They are "semi" in most spheres of their daytime life, and in sleep they lie betwixt the back and the prone positions. In their worlds, they have the ability to get along and to "make do." They are conciliatory in nature and adjust to most situations by compromise and the avoidance of extreme stances. They are best described as middle-of-the-roaders.

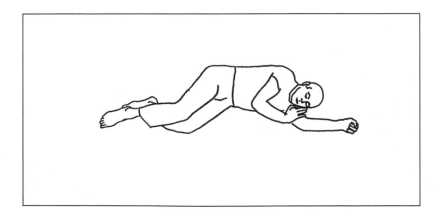

The final basic position is called the Full Fetal, as in the characteristic womb position. These sleepers lie curled on their sides, with knees pulled all the way up, and with their heads bent forward. They usually organize this position around a core pillow or blanket mass. Similarly, in life, they organize their entire being around a significant personal relation, particularly striving for an intense one-on-one involvement, tending to fuse their existences in a close binding symbiosis to a significant other. These sleepers are extremely emotional, sensitive, artistic and have intense one-on-one relationships. Their insomnia is early morning. Women who sleep in this configuration usually have the capacity for multiple orgasms; men show equivalent sexual response patterns.

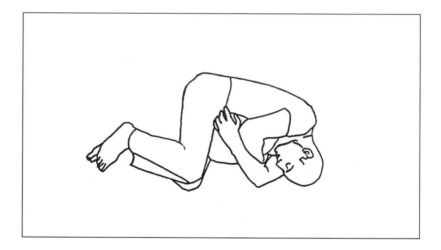

I have noted an interesting correlation with the Full Fetal position. This position seems to be linked with the capacity of women to experience multiple orgasms, an ability, according to Kinsey, experienced by only twelve percent of American women.

These four basic positions are further modified by variations in the attitude of the trunk or the head, and the placement of the extremities. These modulations serve to express wider varieties of individual personality, and often create unusual, picturesque sleep configurations. Many of these variations have been cataloged, and their meanings interpreted in my original work. The evocative names (such as Monkey or Sphinx) used to describe these often exotic individual positions were frequently selected by the persons themselves, or by those who observed their eccentric sleeping postures. The sphinx, that is illustrated, is a common sleep variant. It is seen mainly in children who are oppositional, usually fighting their parents' request to go to bed at a reasonable hour. They are down but not out, still on their knees, resisting the song of the sandman. It is remarkable how long they can sleep in this position until, at last, REM, with its sleep paralysis, brings them down to earth.

There are many other exotic variant sleep positions. A larger catalog is illustrated and in my book *Sleep Positions, the Night Language of the Body*. See notes and references for chapter 15. (Illustrations by Ruth Dunkell.)

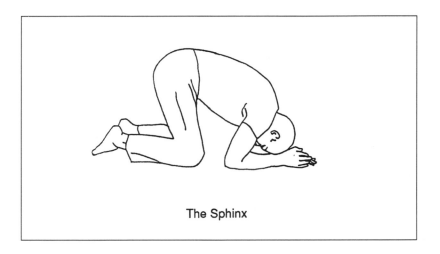

The Sphinx

Alpha and Omega Stages

We fall asleep in two stages. In the first, we lie in bed relaxing with our eyes closed. The brain begins to show spurts of regular, low, rounded EEG (alpha) waves, unlike the agitated, irregular, spiking activity of waking thought. Our body positions in this stage assume the relaxed attitudes of quiet reflection and reverie. These are our Alpha sleep positions. Thinkers, like the philosopher Hannah Arendt, lie recumbent in the Water Wings position, on the back with hands clasped in the rear of the neck and elbows sticking up, in the alpha stage, and seem to be funneling world events into their reflective brains in this quiet preslumber period. Most of us yawn, nod our heads, and show other signs of imminent entry into the sleep world during alpha. It is at this point, as we feel ourselves drifting off into sleep, that we assume our second, or final, Omega position. Our omega position, our most trusted security position, is our actual sleep entry position.

Some sleepers whose personalities are less complex or more rigid than others, may go on to spend most of the night in their alpha position. But most will change to the omega position, the position which gives them the greatest security in preparation for their extended encounter with sleep.

Tokenism of Sleep Positions

If at times we are forced to give up our preferred sleep position, and we find we are unable to fall asleep without it, a compromise is in order. The token use of a small part or body attitude held over from the preferred position, can recapture its security for us when we incorporate it into the new position.

In one well-known literary example of token remembrance, Proust ate a madelaine, a small round sponge pastry, that is commonly consumed with tea in France. This recalled an infinity of past events from his life. A similar process occurs when we practice tokenism in our sleep positions.

Arthritic people sometimes find that their preferred sleep position results in a flare-up of pain that interferes with sleep. As a consequence, they have to make do with a new position which is less painful, but is different from their preferred one. However, they may find themselves unable to sleep in the new unaccustomed position. Tokenism may be the key to recapturing the security of the preferred original position and good sleep.

One royal sleeper, for example, told me that she really preferred to sleep in the prone position, but a back problem forced her to train herself to sleep in the royal position. She was able, though, to retain her feeling of being in the prone position by sleeping with a pillow on her chest. The pillow symbolized the original surface of the bed; its pressure on her chest recalling the prone position. The security of this token reminiscence allowed her to fall asleep easily in this otherwise alien position, and unless she used the pillow in this token way she suffered sleep difficulties.

A particularly striking example of tokenism is illustrated by Ellen

Gerard, a woman in her fifties, who suffered a coronary artery embolism twenty years ago that was caused by the use of contraceptive pills. A full fetal sleeper until that episode, she can only fall asleep now on her back with her upper body raised by pillows. This is reminiscent of the way in which she slept in the hospital while recovering from the heart attack. She sleeps on her back with her head twisted sideways until her cheek rests firmly on the pillows. The cheek contact with the pillow reminds her of her normally preferred side sleep position. The back position and the raised upper body, which reminds her of her hospital position, lets her take out mental insurance against the possibility of a recurrence of the coronary attack.

The most extreme example of tokenism occurs in patients who, following a fracture, are immobilized on their backs in a body cast, with their arms or legs suspended aloft by attachment to a frame over the bed. Even in this abnormal trapezelike position, such individuals are able, through the use of tokenism, to assume their preferred sleep position. They manage to do this by adopting bodily muscle strain patterns within the rigidity of the casts which, in their dynamic configuration, remind them of their basic sleep positions.

Sleep researchers, as mentioned, have become cognizant of the value of utilizing sleep positions in treating sleep apnea, and preventing cot deaths in infants. Sleep position theory is also useful in other branches of medicine, in obstetrics, for example. I have been consulted by women in the later phases of pregnancy who, because of a distended abdomen, find it extremely difficult to fall asleep if they normally prefer to sleep prone. I tell them about tokenism, instructing them to lie on their backs and to tuck toes and hands under the mattress corners. This helps them to adjust to this common difficulty, since it gives them the comforting feeling of control which they had achieved in their prone position. Or, as described earlier, they can achieve the same result by putting a pillow on their chests.

Can Changing Your Sleep Position Change Your Personality?

Since the publication of my work on sleep positions, I have frequently been asked whether changing a sleep position can change your personality. I answer that the reverse is what typically takes place. When you change your everyday behavior in a basic way, then your preferred sleep position will also change, getting into line with your new life position. In my clinical work I have found that the meaning of sleep positions is so graphic and striking, that it can be used as a clue to show you how you can alter a basic life position.

For example, I suggest to full fetal sleepers that perhaps they can open themselves to a broader range of human relationships than their intense one-on-one, frequently stormy, and insomnia engendering attachments. I ask persons who have been shown and apprehend the meaning of the full fetal position to make a polar-opposite transition in their behavior, a full one hundred eighty degree Copernican switch in their life position, rather than in their sleep position, and see what happens as a result. I advise them to try becoming more autonomous, to engage in other, perhaps less intense, emotionally toned types of relationships, and to increase the spectrum and number of personal involvements in their lives.

Or, in another example, I advise the middle-of-the-road semi-fetal sleeper to march to a different drumbeat and adopt more independent positions in life, and then observe what happens with this new approach.

Some royal sleepers cross their arms with their hands covering their chests. This position reveals that although they are generally open people, they still keep a tight control over the existential center of their bodies, the heart area. I ask them to be more completely revealing about themselves, both in therapy and outside of treatment, rather than being seemingly open, yet remaining fundamentally guarded.

A young sleeper whom I treated preferred the prone position. Rather than extending her arms above her head, as is typical in this position, she rested her arms underneath her body, with forearms pinned under her thighs. This position compromised the circulation in her arms, resulting in tingling and sleep-disrupting pain. I mentioned to her that although she seemed to be in a state of extreme control, this imprisoning placement of her arms and hands limited the handling of her environment and had painful consequences for her. I suggested that perhaps it would be wise for her to free herself from this limitation in her active dealings with her world, and to take more initiative in controlling her destiny.

The essence of sleep positions, insomnia patterns, and personality is that they are neither accidental nor mechanical, but rather purposeful, dynamic, and significant. By understanding them, and applying the lessons learned from their meanings, they can help our quest for behavioral change. Overcoming a sleep problem may, at the same time, allow you the opportunity to exert a significant force for improvement in the rest of your life.

Vesuvius and Sleep Positions

In the year A.D. 79 Mount Vesuvius erupted in a mighty series of explosions, overrunning the villages and cities on its surrounding flanks with avalanches of lava. The waves of lava swept down so swiftly that many inhabitants were entombed in their sleep. This event has been memorialized by excavations at the settlements of Pompeii and Herculenium. A large number of sleepers were found to have been perfectly preserved in the lava. Today, the excavated casts of these sleeping citizens can be seen in the Archeological Museum in Naples. The molten silica, created by the enormous temperatures of the volcanic process, served as perfect casting material around the entombed victims, leaving them encased in their exact sleeping positions. The actual configurations demonstrated by these unawakened, eternally entombed sleepers eerily typify the sleeping positions which I described.

The Granny Mystery

Sleep position theory has had some surprising applications. Dr. Ivor Noel Hume, the director of the Colonial Williamsburg Restoration Project in Virginia, brought an interesting one to my attention. On March 22, 1622 a small English settlement in Colonial Virginia was the victim of a sudden Indian attack and massacre. The colonists were killed and scalped, or taken captive and never seen again. After the massacre the dead were buried in the typical burial position of the time, lying on their backs with their hands crossed on their midsections. Their coffins were arranged in regular rows in the ground.

In the excavations at the site, the Williamsburg archeologists found the skeleton of a female adult without a coffin, located some distance away from the other victims. Dr. Hume was puzzled because she was lying in a markedly different position than the others, on her side. Enlightenment came to him when he became ill and, forced to spend some time in bed, became aware of his own semi-fetal sleep position. He suddenly had the insight that the female victim, nicknamed "Granny," must have died, lying where she was found, in a side position similar to the one in which he himself preferred to sleep. Using this insight, he speculated that she might have been partially scalped in the Indian attack and left for dead.

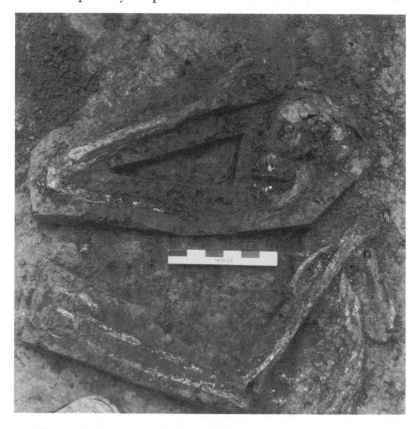

"Granny." (Photo courtesy of Ivor Noel Hume.)

He reasoned further that she may have recovered consciousness and, in attempting to escape, pulled herself to a hiding place in a nearby ravine where, because of exposure and the vulnerability of her wounded state, she perished. The ravine became her tomb, only coming to light in the systematic archeological excavation of the entire area.

In trying to reconstruct and decipher the events of Granny's death, Dr. Hume needed information about sleeping positions. He contacted the State of Virginia's Forensic Offices about the problem and through them was referred to me. An important point made by the forensic experts was that persons dying of exposure experienced a hallucinatory feeling of well-being and warmth shortly before death. It was reasoned that this probably happened to Granny and that in the adverse circumstances of her dying she had settled into her typical sleep position in the hallucinatory pre-death period.

The victim was nicknamed Granny because of the deteriorated condition of her lower molars. In actuality, though, skeletal analysis determined that she was only about thirty-five to forty. Dr. Hume asked me to use my knowledge of sleep positions to speculate about the personality of Granny. The position she assumed was the semi-fetal which, as described, is characteristic of a person who is adaptable and tries to make do. Certainly this type of personality was suited to the rigors of colonialism in the New World, an experience that required a high degree of coping flexibility. I was able to speculate on other aspects of her psychic makeup. A hair band, pushed backward on one side by the scalping, was found on her skull. I thought that the presence of this grooming item indicated that Granny had still maintained her need for personal adornment in the wilderness, showing a strong sense of feminine identity. This case provides an interesting application of the theory of sleep positions in an unexpected area.

Couple Sleep Positions

We have seen that individual sleep positions are consistent with behavior, personality, and emotional state in the day world. Similarly, couple sleep positions reflect the basic behavioral interaction patterns in a couple's relationship. I find it true, also, that if a couple is unable to assume a preferred couple sleep position, either one partner or both suffer sleep difficulties.

The research on sleep is seemingly blinkered in avoiding the reality that most people share a bed with a "significant other." Sleep researchers only seem to take this fact into account when dealing with couple-related sleep difficulties in the limited areas of sleep apnea and sleep behavior disorder; when the interactive presence of more than one person in the bed cannot be overlooked. But in general, the inclination to deal with the abstract isolation of the body, rather than the complex larger life of the person possessing that body, permeates the field of sleep research.

There is a natural history in the evolution of preferred couple sleep positions. The Spoon position is the most common couple sleep position for the first three to five years. In this position, both partners lie on the same side facing in the same direction, one behind the other, like a set of spoons nestled in a drawer. This position allows maximum physical closeness while also showing the emotional closeness of the couple in the early years of their togetherness. Most couples tend to maintain the spoon position for most of the night during this period. When one member turns to the other side, the other follows suit, so that the spoon position is resumed on the opposite side.

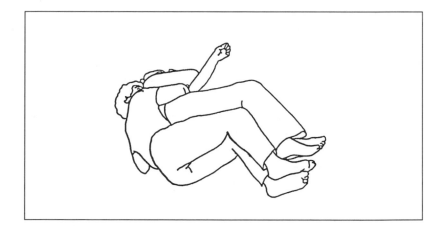

As time goes on, and the security of their relationship is cemented, the two partners may hold the spoon position at the beginning of the night. Then, as the night wears on, they may separate, taking their individual sleep positions while maintaining a sleep reassuring contact through occasional casual touching of extremity or trunk. They may resume the actual spoon position at intermittent periods during the night, and when awakening in the early morning.

An interesting historical note on the spoon position is found in a description of the sleeping circumstances of Union soldiers using the "A-Tent" in the field during the Civil War. "The floor space, some seven feet square was adequate for accommodation of four men; but when six were crowded in, as was frequently the case in the first months of war, soldiers had to sleep 'spoon fashion,' and when one Yank turned over, all had to turn." Through this cooperative sleep effort they were able to maximize their nighttime rest in readiness for the rigors and danger of the day ahead. When one of the soldiers felt he had to turn he would sound off and shout "spoon." Hearing this signal, the others in the tent turned simultaneously, as couples do in their own beds in a semisleep brief awakening during the night.

One of my patients described the spoon position as the small letter "c" surrounded by a large or big "C" with the little "c" person being held by the big "C." This metaphor described her dependency as well as her sexuality. Although she was frequently involved in intense couple relationships, she was so dependent and basically immature, that she admitted never having had the experience of an orgasm in her entire life.

John and Marcy slept in the spoon position until Marcy became pregnant. She was forced to give up this position in the later months of pregnancy when her enlarged abdomen made it impossible for her to sleep in the intimacy of the big "C." Forced by her condition to sleep somewhat apart from John, the loss of her desired close couple sleep position resulted in difficulty in sleeping and she had to consult me for help. I advised the tokenism of a clasped pillow to temporarily "sleep in" for her husband, and as much contact of trunk and legs during sleep as possible for the remainder of her pregnancy. As soon as her pregnancy terminated, she resumed her longed-for spoon position.

A change in the type of bed parallels the process of gradual separation in couple sleep patterns. Over the course of years the beds they use begin to get larger, since more space is needed with the assumption of individual positions. Bed sizes increase from a full size to a queen and eventually to a king. After about twenty years of marriage there is a trend to the use of a Hollywood bed with a single headboard, followed in turn, by adjacent twin beds. Later on, for those having the extra space, separate rooms for him and for her might eventually be used.

Sometimes the drifting apart of the partners in sleep is accelerated by other factors, such as the restlessness of one partner, or the noise of snoring. The problem caused by conflicting sleep schedules, or by the differing preferred lights-out times of larks and owls, might also cause an accelerated separation.

As Groucho Marx once cracked, "It's not politics that makes strange bedfellows. It's marriage."

A young woman described her own sad experience with couple sleep positions to me. During her courtship she had noticed the reluctance of her fiance to enter into close physical contact when they slept together. She made nothing of this, continuing the relationship, which consummated in marriage. Shortly after the marriage, though, she noticed a further intensification of her husband's distancing tendency during sleep. He began to practice the Freeze Maneuver, going to sleep on his side of the bed as far away from her as possible, and turning his back to her during the entire night. His retreat was further emphasized when he took the pillows on which he slept and placed them between himself and his wife.

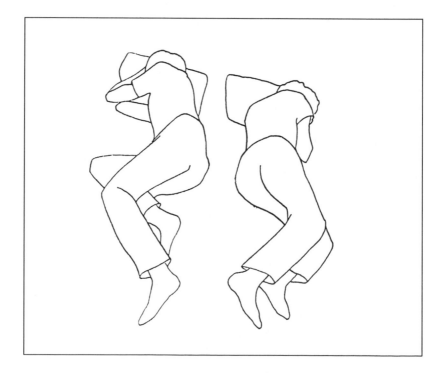

This distancing and barricading in sleep exactly paralleled his puzzling withdrawal from her in the marriage, which shortly thereafter ended in a traumatic separation and divorce. She later learned the reason for his behavior, discovering that he was homosexual and had made an ill-fated attempt at heterosexual life by marrying her. In her interview with me she lamented that if she had known of my work on couple sleep positions and its significance, she might have been more alert and more aware of problems in their early relationship and made a more careful evaluation of the situation before marriage.

Couple sleep positions reflect ongoing interaction patterns. Sleepers who dominate their partners in their daily life tend to continue this power play in bed. The domineering partner may sleep in the Bridge position, placing a leg over the body of the sleeping partner, thereby demonstrating control over the existence of the partner, even in sleep. Usually the royal position is taken by this autocrat. This way of relating is certainly different from the more sharing one seen in the spoon.

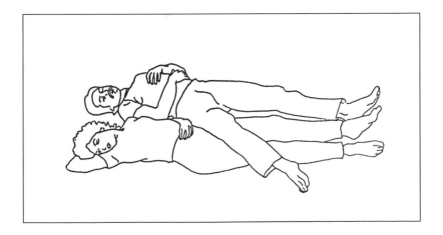

Partners who are overly dependent on their mate often sleep in the Umbilicus position. Their continuing search for security is reinforced in sleep by the tactic of clutching onto the partner, either by placing the hand in a locking position in the partner's armpit, or by placing it between the partner's thighs. Like astronauts floating in space they cannot give up the need for a sustaining secure lifeline, even during sleep.

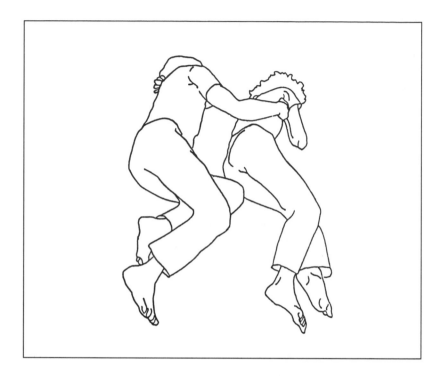

In the Shingle position a partner, usually the male, becomes the image of security and Gibraltarlike stability, lying firmly in the royal position. The dependent and compliant partner also lies on her back, but with her head on the shoulder of her mate. She assumes a security-yielding status by identification. Her position, by overlapping the supporting partner, creates a configuration that resembles shingles on a roof. By looking at the world from the same perspective as her partner, she achieves a strengthening sense of comradeship and protection.

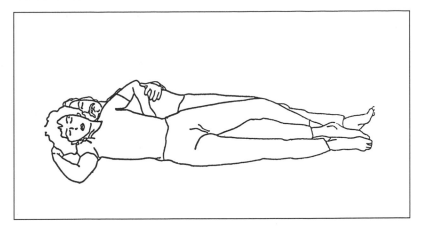

A variation of this position is the Reverse Shingle. In this position one partner lies prone, overlapping the supine other partner. Psychologically, this represents an attempt by the top partner to be entirely absorbed in the other's existence, focusing total attention on the other, even in sleep.

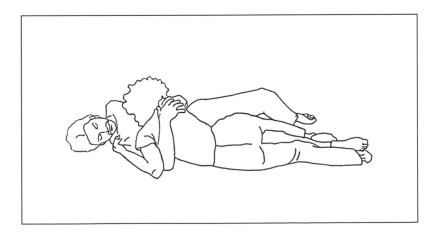

An example of the shingle position was shown by the history of Dorothy Mottley. She had just begun a relationship with a man who was making a serious attempt to form an enduring couple union. In this endeavor, the man insisted that the two of them go to sleep together in the shingle position. Actually, though, at this point in their relationship neither was totally committed to the joining of their existences. This reservation revealed itself in the following sleep pattern. He would usually fall asleep first. Dorothy, who up to this point was unable to sleep, would now turn away from him and slip out of the shingle embrace. Moving to one side of the bed she assumed her preferred sleep position, the semi-fetal, with her back turned to him. He would then, although asleep, turn away from her, and with his back toward her, go into his own sleep position, like hers, in the semi-fetal side position. They would then continue to sleep in these individual positions for the rest of the night.

There was, however, another sleep position which she assumed. I've called this position the Matterhorn; its objective is an attempt at limiting sexual intimacy. Although they spent their weekends together at his country house, they were separated during the work week when Dorothy would return to her job in the city, while he remained in the country. Alone during the week, she discovered herself falling asleep while lying on her back with one knee in the air, in the matterhorn position. Apparently, alone in the city, she was still stimulated emotionally and sexually by their weekends together. She could only relax sufficiently to fall asleep during the weekday hiatus by assuming this position. This enabled her to to shut off the arousing reverie of sexual fantasies, stirred up by their connubial weekends. The raised leg of the matterhorn position reflects her defensive way of limiting her sleep disturbing erotic fantasies, as in actual life, the raised leg would inhibit coitus.

Among the variety of couple sleep positions which I have described are the Hug, the Freeze, the Switch, the Bud, and the Crab.

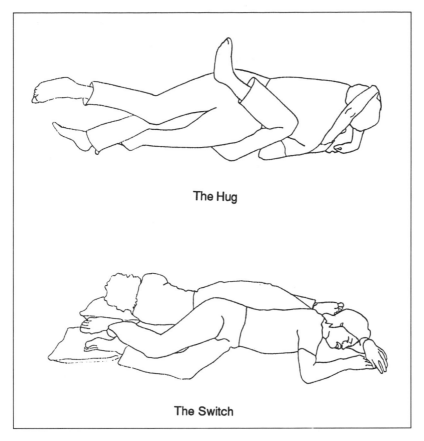

The Hug

The Switch

Sleep in the Tropics—A Case History

My work on sleep positions received wide attention in the media, and as a result of this publicity I received mail from many individuals commenting on their own personal experiences with sleep positions. Of the numerous letters I received, by far the most interesting one came from Rangoon.

1 P.M. Sunday 30 September 1979

Dear Dr. Dunkell,

Sitting in a never ending tropical rainstorm prompted me to pick up a copy of your book *Sleep Positions* from the hotel bookstand. The duration of the rain and the book's inflated local price gave me opportunity and reason to read it twice yesterday and finding an equally wet reception today I thought I would take the opportunity to write to you with some unusual sleep case histories that I hope you might find interesting and useful. Firstly may I congratulate you on producing a most informative and readable book. Secondly may I assure you that this letter is not a request for counselling. Although the three instances that I will tell you about involve myself, I nevertheless consider myself and my partner to be within the parameters of normality. I merely felt that the unusual and possibly unique nature of the three cases may be of some use to you in future works. Lastly, before getting down to brass tacks, it is perhaps important to say that although these cases may indicate an almost laboratory like approach, I had in fact not read anything on the subject of the sleep world until yesterday.

Before going into the three instances in detail I will give you some background on myself and my sleeping partner that may help with interpreting these cases.

I am 26 years old, right handed, my job requires me to often work until 2 A.M. I am a salesman and consequently this goes hand in hand with the frequent consumption of alcohol. I also have a disjointed nose that completely blocks my left nasal passage. As a result of these last two factors I snore! My preferred Alpha position is Water Wing and my predominant Omega position when sleeping alone is Semi-Fetal, on my right side.

My partner for the last 18 months, Shameera, is twenty one. She is also right handed and is a nurse who is often required to do irregular shifts. Her usual Alpha position when sleeping alone is Semi-Fetal on her right side. Her predominant Omega position is Full-Fetal on her right side with a very unusual variation that I will mention later.

I have my own house with a large double bed with its left side against a wall. Shameera lives in an apartment with a single bed that has its right side against a wall. We generally sleep together five or six nights a week in one or the other abode. Because we both work strange shifts either one of us frequently encounters the other already in bed and fast asleep. This gives us ample opportunity to view each other's sleeping habits.

When we are sleeping together our Omega position is predominantly spoons with myself Semi-Fetal, Shameera Full-Fetal and with me in the posterior position.

Now for the cases. . . .

1 My Problem

Ever since I first started sleeping with Shameera, I would wake up in the morning with a stiff neck. It soon became apparent that this stiffness was associated solely with Shameera. On occasions since I had started sleeping with her I had also slept with other women without the resulting neck pain. The pain did not occur when I slept on my own. And even after eliminating all draughts I consistently had the same stiff neck after sleeping with her, irrespective of, if it was at my place, her place or a hotel.

At this time I had read nothing on the sleep world and concluded that I must be contorting the position of my head during sleep thus giving me the resulting pain. But why was it only with Shameera? The situation became so intolerable that I decided to do something about it. I borrowed a low level TV camera and video recording system and set it up to film a complete nights sleep. On viewing the video tape the cause of my problem became immediately apparent.

Shameera had very long and frizzy hair at the time. Often during the twilight period when we would adopt an Alpha Spoon position I would smooth down her hair with my hand to avoid its irritating my face (I am always in the posterior position). It became apparent from the video tape that when I went into the Omega period I would turn my face upwards to avoid this irritation. All the time my torso, arms and legs would remain in the full spoon position. This prolonged twisting of my neck was what I took to be the cause of the stiffness. In retrospect your book has answered one of the puzzles that I was left with after viewing the tape. Most of the time that we were in a spoon position I had my face turned upward but suddenly it would flop back into her hair for prolonged periods without apparently causing me any irritation. Then suddenly I would turn my face upwards again. I now presume that this lapse period was during a paralytic REM phase.

The solution to this problem luckily was very simple. Shameera had often stated that she wanted to have her hair cut into a short, modern style. I had always encouraged her to keep it long as this was my preference and she had always obliged. After finding that her hair had such a profound effect on my sleeping comfort I treated her to the "hair-do" that she had always wanted and overnight the stiffness in my neck disappeared totally. Just imagine, the best prescription for a stiff neck could be a suitable coiffure.

2. Wall Security

As I have already mentioned, my bed has its left side against a wall and Shameera's bed has its right side against a wall. You may also recall that my partner's predominant Omega position is Full-Fetal indicating a degree of insecurity and a desire for protection. Once again we are both right handed.

The interesting factor here is that whether we sleep in my bed or hers, she will always insist on sleeping facing the wall. As this necessitates a right handed person to sleep predominantly on her left side whenever she stays at my place, it would seem contradictory. Yet she seems to be able to maintain this reversed position the following night. More surprising than that is the fact that, when in the Spoon position I can also maintain this reversed posture and equally easily change the following night.

But I think the predominant factor here is the use of the wall. On the odd occasion, out of sheer stubbornness, that I have insisted on sleeping on the inside, my partner has found it impossible to get to sleep. Thus I take it that the wall becomes an extension of the protective content of the Full-Fetal position. Like a scolded child may retreat to a corner for security my sleeping partner is unconsciously demonstrating the same desire to be sandwiched between or be placed as close to a tangible boundary to give her the protectiveness that she requires. A bed situated exactly in the middle of the room may present an interesting dilemma for her subconscious. I may well experiment upon my return.

3, Covered Ears

I notice that in your book you state that you have never come across a case of anyone sleeping with their hands covering their ears. Although some people adopt an Ostrich position using a pillow to block out the sounds of the day world, you feel that they do not use their hands to cover their ears as this is effectively our only early warning system in the sleep world.

Once again, Shameera, my sleeping partner, has proved an exception to the rule. On many occasions that I have arrived at her apartment late and found her already asleep I have noticed that she has one or both hands covering her ears. Sometimes she goes to the extent of putting her index fingers into her ears. I first noticed this one night that I woke up prematurely and found her in this position three or four hours after she went to sleep. When I asked her why she thought that she did it she said it was to block out the noise of my snoring. This, however, does not explain why she should do it before I arrive.

I had also noticed that on occasions that she did this she also talked in her sleep and appeared to be having nightmares. Shameera is not English and consequently when she talks in her sleep she reverts back to her native language. Unfortunately I do not speak this language so her mutterings offer me no clue as to what she is dreaming about. The following morning she has no knowledge of the content of her nightmares and generally cannot even remember having them. Puzzled?

I think the cause of this unusual ear covering and her need to get close to walls may be explained by her background. When Shameera was fifteen or sixteen she underwent a traumatic experience. Her whole family were expelled from her home and country overnight by a despotic regime. In addition to this when she was ten or eleven, perhaps in early puberty, she spent about a year in a war zone in Bangladesh that underwent quite heavy shelling and bombardment. I would imagine that a psychologist would consider this a classic recipe for insecurity and give rise to a need for protection.

I wonder, could it be that her nightmares are about her experiences in Bangladesh, and the fact that she covers her ears could be a subconscious attempt to block out the noise of the shelling, as she probably did in her day world experiences at that time.

Well I hope you found this information interesting. If you do require any further information on these instances I would be happy to supply it. In the event that you are going to reply to this letter I would appreciate it if you would let me know of any other books you have written on this subject or any future works that you have planned. A short suggested bibliography of the sleep world would also be appreciated.

Yours sincerely,
E. W.

* * *

Knowing the meanings of sleep positions, including couple sleep positions, is of great value in psychotherapy sessions. It is especially significant in couple counseling, where such meanings, when spelled out, can be enlightening to the troubled pair. I find that if the couple sleeps in the spoon position, despite the presence of conflict in other aspects of their relationship the prognosis is positive for a good outcome to the counseling intervention.

It is important in couple sleep—as in individual sleep positions—to state that no value judgments in interpretations are made. There are no best, or recommended, or ideal sleep positions, just as there are no best amounts of sleep length. Sleep position analysis, in correlation with evaluations of the prevailing emotional and personality patterns, simply allows us to better understand the relationships that exist in couple situations without being laudatory or pejorative about them.

For example, two partners in a couple relationship may be somewhat detached in their individual personalities and prefer a certain degree of aloofness and distance in human relationships. This distancing tendency may show itself in their sleep positions by an avoidance of physical closeness in sleep. Owing to their personality needs this mode of interaction is an optimum one for them, both individually and as a couple. Such emotional and physical coolness is part of the basic, unwritten couple contract to which they have subscribed, and an important feature of their partnership and of their sleep arrangement.

A special circumstance is presented when the ongoing preferred mode of a couple sleep position changes abruptly, or relatively suddenly. When one partner, or both, suddenly adopt a freeze maneuver (turning the back to the bed partner and at the same time moving away in bed), or other distancing tactics, it is an indication that a difficulty in the partnership arrangement is causing the withdrawal during sleep. As in individual sleep position analysis, such sudden changes can yield excellent clues as to the direction that remedial action can take. In the case of the bridge position (dominating the partner by crossing a leg over the partner's lower limbs and pinning the partner down), for example, it often happens that the more compliant partner begins to seek more autonomy and equality in the relationship. The goals of therapeutic action are clearly indicated by the couple's sleep positions. The dominating and power-seeking consort should attempt to give up the controlling attitude and allow the submissive partner to get out from under. At the same time the formerly docile partner should strive for more independence and more self-direction.

* * *

The plastic nature of sleep positions reveals not only our enduring personality traits, but also reflects more transient defensive needs, for example, Shameera's covering her ears during the course of the night. Another instance of this flexibility occurred in the case of a woman who was resisting a painful insight in her psychotherapy. She demonstrated this defensiveness at night by assuming a position during sleep with her hand covering her eyes. This posture was maintained despite the extreme discomfort she felt when she awoke, due to the pressure of her hand on her eyes.

Psychological security needs show themselves not only on going to bed—as in the major sleep positions we ordinarily assume at lights-out time—but in our sleep behavior throughout the night. Clinical anecdotes like this verify the existence of the ever present interplay of body and mind in sleep.

Chapter 16

Intimacy

Although sleep and death—the so-called "Big Sleep"—are often linked, there is another common correlation, the equation of sleep and love. We can see this in the use of such terms as "to go to bed," "to lie down with one another," "to get laid," and "to sleep with someone" as synonyms for love and sex. Associating sleep with a feeling of emotional closeness seems natural to us. In fact, the phrase "lying in the arms of Morpheus" to personify sleep, clearly expresses the connection between sleep and intimacy. To "become intimate with someone" usually means having sex and going to bed with that person.

There are many reasons why we think of intimacy in connection with sleep. Sleep is a nocturnal event and, whereas the days are for activity and work, our nights are for rest and intimacy.

Preoccupation with the struggles of daily life is put aside. Rest and relaxation become the focus of our beings. Time pressure is absent. We have the feeling that there is a blank space in the day until the alarm goes off in the morning.

Although we attempt to eliminate the distracting stimulation of the day world from the bedroom, we admit those elements in the environment which increase intimacy, security, and release. Soporific sounds—like the soft, rhythmic patter of rain on the roof, the rustle of trees or bushes, subdued urban sounds, or the muted ringing of church bells in early morning—may be part of the sleep scene.

The nighttime hiatus, with its serenity and loss of definition of far-off things, allows us to refocus on our bodily needs, emotional expression, and intimacy.

We quiet down as bedtime approaches; stillness is a precondition for sleep. This stillness adds to our sense of intimacy by allowing us to concentrate on one another, shutting out the distractions of external demands. Talk is subdued. What one partner has to say is only meant for the other's ears—it is an "intimate communication."

Relaxation and lack of restraint go together. Perhaps sixty percent of the American public sleep in the nude. Those who wear nightgowns, pajamas, or underwear, find they sleep best when these are large and loose; giving them a feeling of being unfettered in sleep, and the ability to move around in bed freely and unbound.

With relaxation, ease, security, and a sense of a coming renewal, there is a natural tendency to review the day's activities at bedtime. This review takes the form of "pillow talk," an intimate communication characterized by confidentiality, mutuality, and the abandonment of guardedness and defensiveness. For these reasons, it is no accident that popular myth has Mata Hari using the bedroom as her arena for espionage.

The horizontal position in bed removes the need to consider the environment since, in effect, attention is directed only at an unbounded heaven with its promise of infinity. This is true even though heaven is represented by the plain plaster ceiling of the bedroom.

Being alone together, and close to one another in the muted void, accentuates our feelings of oneness and intimacy. Lying down removes the need to overcome the pull of gravity; bringing relaxation to body and mind. Since most of us enter the sleep world every day with the same partner, the feeling of familiarity further enhances intimacy and security.

Sharing a bed and bedroom tends to inhibit aggressive behavior. It is difficult for us to relax when aroused or on guard. This is why we attempt to iron out disagreements before going to sleep. Our physical and emotional contact with another person in the close quarters of the bed dispels loneliness, inspires security, and allows us to unwind and let down all our guards. The warmth of the partner's body recalls, on some level, the closeness to the security-giving person of the earliest stages of life, the mother. The swaddling effect of bedcovers enhances such feelings.

We become aware of vital functions, such as the pulsation of the heartbeat, when we sleep close to our bedmate; figuratively, we are in touch with his or her center of being. In the bed and bedroom we experience our partner in all basic, physical, emotional, and intimate aspects. When nightmares and anxiety-provoking dreams diminish security feelings, closeness and protection are called for. The partner's presence gives the frightened dreamer reassurance and strength. Sharing toileting and hygiene, we are unguarded—without daytime makeup, clothing, disguises, secrets, or shame. The coolness of an optimum sleep environment also encourages physical closeness, with partners clinging together for warmth. The intimacy of love is not only heightened by the convenience of the horizontal position and its comforts, but other factors are available to stimulate intimacy and eroticism.

Psychological research has made us aware of the importance of touch for human security. The need for touch between lovers and bed partners underscores this sort of intimacy, especially in the early stages of the couple relationship. Touching stimulates skin eroticism, which heightens the need for closeness and the desire for intimacy. There is an affinity between our sense of security, and eroticism and touch.

The closeness of couple sleep positions allows maximum skin contact of highly erotic areas. Arousal takes place during REM periods and is most frequent in the late night–early morning hours, because of the increase in REM at these times. This accounts for males frequently awakening with morning erections, and corresponding genital responses occurring in women. The effects of REM genital arousal at these times may stimulate erotic activity. Experiments involving the theory of affiliation have shown that there is a search for physical and emotional contact as well as an increase in erotic fantasy, in situations involving arousal.

Sleep Discord

Despite the favorable factors in the sleep world that enhance relaxation, openness, sharing, intimacy, and eroticism, all may not go well in the bedroom. The result can mean interference with sleep. Discordant notes are sounded only too often in the night.

Problems arise when sleepers have different preferences for room temperature during the night. When conflict over preferred temperature is a problem a good solution might be twin beds pushed together, with separate amounts of bed covers.

For differences in sleep timing between a lark and an owl, the late retiring owl can try getting into bed with the early-to-bed lark at lights-out time until the lark is asleep, then quietly get out of bed. Conversely, a lark should understand the night owl's difficulties with awakening in the morning.

When one partner is an imperialist, moves more than the other and pushes the other to an uncomfortable edge-of-the-bed position, the solution might be a larger bed, or twin beds.

Sensitivity about being touched during the night can be a source of conflict. Some people like to cuddle, whereas others are averse to being touched because it interferes with their sleep. When a partner with high cuddling needs feels rejected if the sleepmate shies away, a loving partner will try to emphasize intimacy, closeness, and love during waking hours, to make up for the distance he or she prefers in sleep.

Some insomnia sufferers cannot sleep in the same bed, or even in the same room, with another person. The discomfort is so intense if such separation proves impossible, their reactions resemble a phobic response. Sometimes conflicted persons try to overcome their fears, and gamble on sharing a bed for a night or so with a lover. The undertaking usually ends negatively. Moreover, the anxiety caused by the attempt may be so great that it is followed by a rebound aversion against ever again trying to share a bed with anyone! This will be reinforced if the love experience is associated with a rejection by the partner, or even if, for whatever reason, it ends on a conflicted problematic note. The situation may be so negative it will cause a conditioned insomnia, even when sleeping alone thereafter.

Insomnia is a very important factor in diminished intimacy. The insomniac does not want closeness in many cases, since he or she is concerned with the freedom and ability to relax at bedtime and, as a result, views sexual and emotional demands for closeness as an interference in being able to fall asleep.

Sexual drive is lowered when persons are depressed, but is heightened during a manic episode. Some manic individuals regularly have intercourse three or four times a night during their high periods and this, of course, may cause significant sleep disturbance for a repeatedly awakened partner.

The nightmarish effects of rapid eye movement (REM) rebound, associated with the use of REM suppressant drugs in depression, as well as in chronic alcoholism and substance abuse, may create such a high degree of anxiety when it occurs that it may interfere with sexual capacity. The resulting sexual inhibition may cause friction with the sexually nonincapacitated partner. As a consequence, the frustrated partner may show reactive rage and aggressive behavior.

Insomnia itself may be related to problems in sexual functioning. In fact, insomniacs are less likely to be married than the general population. Does this mean that insomnia causes sex difficulties which prevent marriage? This data must be viewed with care, since it is possible that the insomnia is a result of the single person's psychological difficulties rather than the cause. Psychological conflicts and interpersonal difficulties interfere with sleep capacity through their stress effects.

A conflict ridden relation can make orgasm impossible or result in other dysfunctional behavior in women; in men, it may cause impotence or retarded ejaculation. Sleep is disturbed for both partners by such distress.

Kinsey, commenting on the correlations of sexual stimulation with sleep, reported that a number of women who were highly aroused by sex found it difficult to fall asleep. He also recognized that whereas some individuals responded to orgasm with arousal, others became fatigued and sleepy. When unable to achieve orgasm, both men and women suffer uncomfortable genital and pelvic blood vessel engorgement, causing tension that leads to disturbed sleep. Sex may be used as a soporific. Some insomniacs attempt to overcome sleep difficulties by masturbation or intercourse at bedtime, or when awakened during the night and unable to return to sleep.

When a conflicted couple relationship has a down side for intimacy, sharing is diminished in extent and quality. For example, partners may go to sleep at different times, leading to a decrease in emotional and physical contact.

Distancing may also be associated with negative off-putting sleep positions, such as the freeze. Such physical contact as remains may be compromised by its contentious nature and aggressive intent. Pushing away, striking, or egocentric imperialism in the bed can occur. Intimacy is disturbed when a sleeper dons scratchy or woolly bedclothing as armor to repel an amorous partner's advance. Coolness in the bed is accentuated by separate covers and by placing pillows far apart. Pillows may be used to create a Maginot Line in bed for similar purposes. There can even be a distancing demand for separate beds or bedrooms. Intimacy is inhibited by a partner's physical condition, such as cold feet, snoring, and restlessness.

Insomniacs are sensitive to the sounds and movements of a sleep partner. Since they worry about sleep, and also have the tendency to become hyperaware of the world and its problems, their thought focus is glued to the day's conflicts. The result of this fixation is an arousal that prevents them from closing their eyes, shutting out the world, and being able to sleep. This preoccupation with the day and its problems also inhibits their readiness for intimacy at night.

When a person suffers from a physical illness such as arthritis, peptic ulcer, a cardiovascular disorder, or breathing difficulties, the physically troubled individual tends to shy away from physical intimacy and retreats into self-absorption.

It is important for partners to remove those barriers that separate them in bed, as in life. Increasing the time spent together, and sharing activities that both enjoy, are helpful in overcoming impediments to intimacy.

Friction should be aired if it arises, and partners should try to recognize and maturely accept the special sleep needs of the other.

Bedrooms and Insomnia—Two Settings

The bed and bedroom are closely identified with our own persona. We are most secure in our own homes, and even more so in our own beds. Bedrooms reflect our nature by including photographs, mementos, designs, and other representations which express our identities. Our preferences in coloration, lighting, types of materials, bed coverings, and sizes of the rooms or beds also call attention to our individuality.

In the late 50s, and even into the 60s, some of my patients reported a special correlation of bedroom, insomnia, and sexuality. They described two different types of sleep environments associated with their early years which later led to sleep and sexual difficulties.

In one, an urban milieu, they grew up in a "railroad flat." This was an architectural floor plan common in low-rise houses and private dwellings of the time. There were no hallways in this layout and one room opened up directly into another, like cars in a railroad train. Bedrooms were located next to each other and very often the parents' bedroom was only separated from the child's by a thin glass doorway, or a curtained archway.

It was interesting to me to see that this structural motif was also carried out in nineteenth century Mittel-Europa buildings. In this architectural style, a building was constructed around a central courtyard and rooms were contiguous to one another. Thus to go from one bedroom to another, it was necessary to traverse the other sleeping quarters. When I happened to look at the floor plan of Sigmund Freud's apartment, at Berggasse 19 in Vienna, I noticed that the apartment was laid out on this model, and it appears that Minna Bernays, Freud's sister-in-law, had to go through the Freuds' master bedchamber in order to reach her own room. She lived with the Freud family most of her adult life and Freud took many vacations traveling alone with her. The intimacy of their sleep lives adds even more questions to the many speculations about their relationship.

To return to my point: Because of the closeness and lack of privacy in this setting, many young children grew up highly aware of their parents' lovemaking by hearing the sounds emanating from their parents' nearby bedroom. I've noticed the strong impact of these experiences in the histories of many patients. Not only did these experiences leave behind a legacy of conflicted psychological states, but they also caused a childhood insomnia which, I believe, often carried over into a later adult insomnia.

I mentioned the urban setting first. The other pattern was seen in patients brought up in rural areas in Europe, particularly in places where entire families slept together over the hearth.

Although a history of sleeping together is credited by some authors with helping to foster security, it sometimes resulted, in patients whom I have encountered—like the railroad flat cases—in later childhood and adult insomnia patterns, as well as protracted neurotic conflicts. I stress that these circumstances were historically limited, since urban architectural practices have obviously changed, as have living conditions in agricultural societies.

The Sentinel Function

An opposite pattern also exists. Some people can only sleep when they are with someone else who grants them the necessary sense of being on guard, and its concomitant feeling of security, that allows them to fall and stay asleep. The partner assumes a sentinel role and continues "on duty," not only at the beginning of sleep, but throughout the night.

Mary Columbo's sleep as a child became conditioned to the presence of the people who gave her a feeling of security. Like many children, she was unable to fall asleep until her parents came home at night.

Mary was a Mafia princess who grew up as the darling of her gangster father. His underworld activities required him to be out at all hours of the night. In her later life, as well as in her childhood, she was unable to sleep until her beloved father, and later her father substitutes, returned home to share her presleep period, allowing her to relax enough to enter the sleep world. Unfortunately, as so often happens in these scenarios, her mobster father was "rubbed out" in a gangland execution. This event caused the onset of a severe chronic insomnia which followed her throughout her later life.

Mary married at a young age and was able to counteract her insomnia with a husband who satisfied her sleep sentinel requirement. Their subsequent separation and divorce, as well as other conflicts, caused such a severe depression and intractable insomnia that she required hospitalization. Her depression was alleviated in the hospital with antidepressants, but her insomnia remained intact.

We were able to uncover the existing sentinel need during the course of her insomnia treatment. As a result of this enlightenment, short term focused psychotherapy was able to help her to overcome her chronic sleeplessness and to dispense with the need for a sentinel in her bedroom.

The dynamics of the sentinel function are shown very clearly in the case history of Elizabeth Chargin who also grew up adoring her father. She was his favorite child. As in Mary Columbo's history, the father came home late, after work, and she stubbornly stayed awake until he arrived and played with her. This idyllic childhood romance was interrupted by the divorce of her parents. After the divorce the patient's mother took her to live with an uncle who, like her father, loved her, and served as a substitute good father figure. He lived on a ranch where she learned to ride, developing a lifelong love of horses. She always insisted upon owning horses in her adult life. She lived in exurban and semirural areas in order to have a barn and grounds where she could keep her cherished horses.

The need for a father figure also persisted, and it followed that she married a powerful man who, she thought, would take the place of her omnipotent father and uncle figures. Owing to her psychological conflicts—which involved very strong oedipal elements—she suffered from a phobic fear that intruders would break into her home while she slept and rape her. This phobia, a torment to her in her single life, found relief in her marriage. Her husband was a poor sleeper, whose restlessness kept him awake a large part of the night. With him she slept like a babe back in her father's arms. He was awake to guard against imagined threatening intruders and rapists! He performed marvelously in his sentinel function.

Fate, once again, was against her since the marriage had much friction and terminated in divorce. Shortly thereafter, luckily, the patient was able to remarry.

Her new husband had a personality which was exactly the opposite of her first mate and apparently was a corrective for his abrasiveness. He was placid, agreeable, and somewhat passive, where her first husband had been irritable, argumentative, and aggressive. The new relationship was a compatible and pleasant one. The sudden development of severe insomnia was an unexpected event.

The new situation in the bedroom was utterly opposite to the one with the first husband. Her second partner was a profound, hypersomniac sleeper, falling asleep rapidly and sleeping deeply for long periods. In addition, he was somewhat deaf and difficult to awaken. When she would desperately shake him awake during her midnight panics, he would grope for his glasses and it took some time for him to become alert and attentive to the external world. She had lost the security of a precious sentinel, the guardian of her sleep, and was forced to take over this function herself, spending practically all night listening anxiously for intruders, and unable to relax and fall asleep. Since the couple needed a barn for her horses, they lived on an isolated farm, which added to her fears and problems. There were no people in the immediate vicinity, no policemen on the beat, no cab drivers and pedestrians, who could have afforded her some security in the nighttime.

Eventually, in near despair, Elizabeth sought treatment for her insomnia. In the process, the treatment included work with her husband as well. In couple therapy they were able to overcome the frictions which had arisen as a result of her anger toward him for failing to serve as guardian of her sleep. Focused individual psychotherapy gave her insights into the true causes of her sleep problem. She was able to deal with the psychological roots of her insomnia and overcome her phobic fears so that unguarded sleep became possible for her at last.

Chapter 17

Gender and Sleep

Pregnancy, Sleep, and Dreams

Some problems in sleep are specifically related to gender. Pregnancy is accompanied by sleep changes. Women nap during early pregnancy and fall asleep more easily than usual, sleeping more deeply and for longer periods. The increase in sleep adds up to an extra two hours per night. This increased sleepiness begins to recede as the second trimester approaches, with a gradual return to normal levels.

Waking tendencies, and problems in falling back to sleep, increase as pregnancy advances. A study showed that thirteen percent of women had sleep difficulties in the first trimester. This figure rose in the second and reached sixty-six percent by the end of the third trimester. In the fifth month, the beginning of fetal movements, and the concomitant psychological conflicts that may occur at this time, cause a notable but transient increase in sleep difficulty.

Body changes in later stages cause women to lose sleep. There is an increase in urinary pressure, because of uterine enlargement, which results in sleep interruption. This enlargement has other effects. The comfort of a preferred sleep posture is jeopardized, as we saw in the case of the pregnant woman who had to give up her preferred spoon position. Changes in body size and shape may cause a woman psychic conflict over her disturbed body image. And fetal kicks and movements reach a crescendo as term nears.

Employed mothers-to-be stop working by the ninth month. This gives them the opportunity to take more daytime naps to offset the increased sleep disruption.

Most difficulties during pregnancy seem to be caused primarily by physical discomfort, although psychological factors may play a role. This can be deduced by the evidence of dream contents in pregnancies. Although most dreams have themes of fertility, there are also dreams that show fears of miscarriage. Dream motifs of danger and intrusiveness emerge when there are conflicts about the pregnancy. Some dreams may also relate to body image, reflecting the changes in shape created by pregnancy. Fears of lifestyle changes occur often. Fears about labor, and changes in relationship to the husband and to her own parents, are typical in late pregnancy.

* * *

Jane S. was having troubles in her second marriage. It was at this time that she discovered she was pregnant. Since she was well into her adult years her obstetrician suggested amniocentesis—a new and experimental procedure at that time—to check for the possibility of Down's syndrome. Anxiously arriving for her test at the medical center, Jane eventually found herself lying on an examining table in a space age setting, surrounded by mysterious electronic equipment. The attending doctor was called away for a telephone call as she was being prepared for the procedure, and she lay alone in this alien environment, with mounting fear, for a relatively long period until the doctor's return rescued her.

A few months later, in the last third of her pregnancy, Jane began to have nightly dreams of hearing a telephone bell ringing. The ringing was so real to her that she would get out of bed and go to the bedroom door in her sleep, awakening to find herself looking down the corridor. This repetitive dream was obviously a rerun of the trauma of the amniocentesis experience. In her own bedroom, she tried to overcome the stress of lying on the laboratory table in terror by arising from her bed to look for the rescuing doctor, as she had not been able to do at the medical center. The sleepwalking parasomnia disappeared by merely explaining to her that her experience of the return of a recent anxiety was not an unusual occurence under the stress of the last trimester.

* * *

Sleep worsens in the immediate aftermath of delivery. Women are wakeful during the first postpartum night, but sleep disturbances diminish rapidly the following nights and sleep patterns return to normal in about two to three weeks, although occasionally this may take as long as six weeks.

Shifts in the new mother's wake–sleep schedules caused by an infant's care and feeding sometimes account for the beginning of a protracted insomnia problem.

Menopause and Sleep

Sleep in women changes with advancing age. However, these age connected changes, and the sleep difficulties they bring with them, do not take place as rapidly in women as in men, lagging ten years behind. It is not until the eighth decade that the incidence of sleep problems becomes equal in men and women. There is a dramatic change in the perimenopausal period. The prevalence of insomnia in women goes from thirty-six percent at the age of thirty to fifty percent at the age of fifty-four, presumably the result of meno-pausal changes and their physical and psychological effects on sleep.

Studies which attempt to correlate the relationship between dream themes and the hormonal changes in a woman's menstrual cycle show interesting, but sometimes confusing, results. Manifest sexual dream themes were highest during menses in a number of surveys, and seemed to be correlated with the increase in estrogen production in the preovulatory phase.

Nocturnal Penile Tumescence

In men, penile erections accompany REM sleep and occur at all ages, from the cradle to the grave. Erections associated with dream periods occur as early as two to four months after birth. At the other end of the age spectrum, it has been demonstrated that men in their nineties have normal patterns of erection, with only a min-imal decrease in penile rigidity, during REM sleep.

One of the many valuable results of sleep research has been the development of tests which discriminate between impotence of an organic nature (commonly caused by diabetes, vascular, and other physical problems) and the impotence that comes from psychic conflicts. Erection is absent when there is an organic problem, but occurs during REM when the impotence is psychological.

Some men believe they are impotent when, in reality, they are not. The "pseudoimpotence" can be discounted by checking on actual states of erection in REM during testing. Most men referred to sleep laboratories are sent for this diagnostic purpose. REM erection, known as Nocturnal Penile Tumescence (NPT), is measured in the laboratory in four ways: by frequency; circumference; duration; and by quality (the degree of penile rigidity). Middle-aged males have three maximum erections during REM in an average night, with each episode of erection lasting approximately twenty-five minutes.

Psychological influences seem to have little direct effect on penile erections during REM sleep, although dream anxiety causes some indirect, minimal variability in circumference.

Chapter 18

Dreamlands

"We are such stuff as dreams are made on" wrote Shakespeare. The proposition that dreams were revelations of the Gods prevailed in the ancient world. By the Middle Ages, though, dreams had lost their divine nature and were thought to be manifestations of humanity's own experiences and attitudes. In this environment, dream books—which interpreted dreams—came into vogue. The rationalists of the eighteenth century considered dreams to be expressions of bodily functions. Romantic poets and thinkers of the nineteenth century returned to a more spiritual account, but beginning late in the century, with the burgeoning of technology and science, there was a revival of the concept that dreaming was a psychological distillation of physical processes occurring during sleep.

Modern psychological theories of the dream began at the same time as the twentieth century, with the publication of Freud's *Interpretation of Dreams* in 1900. The pivotal discovery at midcentury in 1953, of REM sleep and its later correlation with dreaming, opened up new avenues for the study of the phenomenon of dreaming.

Nature of Dreams

We have few memories of our voyage through the night aside from occasionally waking during sleep. The major exceptions are dreams. Consciousness or thought does not stop in sleep. It is merely expressed in another form. The forms of sleep thinking, though, are different from those of daytime consciousness, being more "hallucinatory" and not tied to the conditions of our everyday reality. When this thinking has a narrative quality and is more than just simple images or thoughts, and has complexity and a scenario structure that moves forward in a storylike way, then we label this sleep thinking experience a dream.

Dreaming does not only occur at night, however. We are all familiar with the daydream. In daydreaming we turn inward and try to diminish contact with the external world. Similarly, as we go to sleep the same thing takes place. At first we lose control over the flow of thought. Our thinking wanders and goes its own way, liberated by a loss of orientation to clock time and the mundane geography of the daytime space which we inhabit. Our thinking, at this point, is no longer tied to an external reality that disappears, as, unaware, we are cast adrift in a sea of dreams.

Dreams differentiate themselves from daytime thought and reveries by several important features. Scenes change rapidly. People from the past appear in the present. We are not free in our dreams but are captured by our imagined scripts and are usually unable to willfully direct our thoughts. This characteristic has been described as "single-mindedness." We feel alone in a bizarre universe, finite but unbounded, from which we cannot step back or take distance, and which we, without surprise or protest, placidly accept. Emotions are more important than logical processes in dreams.

Though excited by sexual encounters, the actual poignancy of sexual feelings are absent in dreaming. Absent also is the barbed experience of pain. Dreams may be clear and sharp, or fuzzy. We may appear as actors in our dreams, or we may be looking on at ourselves, or just experience the dream like detached observers, much as we do with personally irrelevant movies or TV shows.

Dream Recall

Most dreams occur during REM, with several different dreams occurring in each REM episode. Given the usual four to five REM periods per night, we all have about twenty different dreams during our night of sleep. Most of us, however, only recall one or two in a week. Freud assumed that dreams are meant to be forgotten, and that the dream in some way is the protector of sleep, allowing it to continue without the danger of our being awakened by anxious thought.

Some people remember more dreams than others. If we are awakened during a dream, or some minutes after it has stopped, it may be remembered. Research shows that training in recalling dreams, as well as a presleep intention to remember, helps recall them. Rapid awakening after a dream also helps its recall, since this gives time for daytime consciousness to imprint the recently experienced dream before it begins to fade. For this reason light sleepers who awaken quickly are better at remembering than heavy sleepers. Nonrecallers tend to be deniers and repressors in their personalities. People who are more facile in recalling dreams, such as long sleepers, seem more open to ambiguity and psychological awareness.

The nature of the dream may play a role in its recall. Dreams that are disturbing have a tendency to be remembered. Vivid dreams make a stronger imprint and are more easily recollected.

Since a greater amount of REM takes place nightly in childhood and diminishes with age, it follows that dreams are more frequent in youth and early adulthood, decreasing in number after the age of fifty.

The special quality of bizarreness in dreams has its origin in changes in identity, unusual plots, strange feelings, discontinuities, and in an unusual matching of circumstances and things. This feeling of looking through a glass darkly is increased by the typical transmutations of persons, animals, and objects, adding to the baroque quality. Bizarreness diminishes as we age; dreams in the later years tend to be more muted. Since one-third of our life is spent in sleep and twenty-five percent of this time is spent in REM, it follows that one-tenth of our lifetime is spent dreaming. There is more REM toward the end of a night's sleep and we tend, therefore, to dream more toward the morning. Dreams also become more "dreamlike" in their bizarreness and complexity at this time, functioning like reprises in the climactic last movements of symphonies.

Most of our dreams are remembered as occurring in black and white. Research has shown this to be incorrect; most dreams actually are in color. Color quality in dreams is evanescent, though, having a tendency to fade away. Dreams take place at the actual speed of the events they portray. There is no fast forward button in dreaming. Although we are functionally blind and each eye goes its own way incoordinately in the rest of sleep, our eye movements during REM become consensual again, both moving effectively together as a unit. Eye movements follow the action of a dream. If we ascend stairs, the eyes move stepwise upward. If we dream we are watching a tennis match, the eyes bounce back and forth in the horizontal plane.

The Senses in Dreams

The most active sense in dreaming is the visual. Do blind people dream? No. Not if they have been blind from birth. Not in pictures, that is. A blind patient of mine, when asked to describe her dreaming and her perception of others in dreams, said that in dreaming she sensed people as the presence of a mass, much as she felt them physically in her day world, without a visual perception of the appearance of a person.

For those individuals who become blind later in life, dreams do have visual images. As they get older, however, there is a tendency for the amount of visual dreaming to diminish, as though the store of these images was being used up.

The other senses that are present in dreams, in order of prevalence, are the auditory, followed by body position and temperature, then touch and, least frequently, smell and taste. The latter two occur in only one percent of all dream phenomena.

When speech occurs in dreams, it usually does not originate with a character but is merely heard, as on an accompanying sound track, without being associated with a particular speaker.

The emotions that occur in dreams are most often anxiety and surprise. Anger is relatively infrequent, occurring in nine to fourteen percent of dreams.

Functions of Dreams

Some dream theorists regard dreams as having a parallel existence with waking life, merely transferring the reality of our daytime existence to a different dimension. Others see dream experience as having an independent, autonomous life of its own. Many writers on dreams cite the effects of day activities on dream events, stressing the causal relationship between events in the day world and those which follow in the night world. The idea that diet will influence dreaming is a common derivative of this view. Eating foods that are spicy or difficult to digest is said to be followed by an increase in dream production and unpleasant dreams. Sleep researchers debunk this view. They believe that the indigestion that follows indulgence causes more awakening which increases dream recall.

Drugs taken during the day or in the presleep period can also influence dreaming, because of their effects on REM. Those which inhibit REM are followed by later REM rebound, which produces more dreams, with more vividness, nightmarishness, and recall capacity. The alcoholic's dreamlike state of delirium tremens is now interpreted as caused by alcohol withdrawal and its associated intense REM rebound effect.

The function of dreams is also considered to be complementary to waking life, supplementing or compensating for distressing daytime experiences. In this way they bring redress and balm to our existence, allowing us to regain psychic balance. They smooth the raveled sleeves of life and help keep us upbeat. Dreams also enable us to look at things from fresh perspectives, unlocking opportunities for other ways of dealing with difficult life experiences.

Dreams fulfill the psychological need of ego strengthening and repair of our frayed self-esteem. The freedom of dream thinking enables us to deal with stressful situations and metabolize them psychologically in order to ensure emotional stability.

Creativity is an important need for humans. In viewing our problems and activities from new perspectives beyond the limiting framework of the day world, dreams allow us to approach problems and activities in another way; giving us a greater freedom of imagination with its ability to resolve conflicts. The regressive aspects of dreaming, and the greater freedom of emotionality in dreams, permit life's spontaneous and playful elements to flourish, nourishing our imagination and creativity.

In a study, the sequence of dreams during the course of a night was charted by waking the dreamers during each successive REM period. It was found that the dream themes at different stages of the night relate to one another and represent a consistent effort to deal with a specific problem. The first dream period, like the statement of a leitmotif, introduces the theme. The next dream periods attempt to relate the theme to our past, especially in terms of stored experiences which have similar emotional significance. The last dreams of the night are pointed toward the future in terms of possible ways out. The emotions connected to the potential consequences of the reality situations, are held at a low pitch in this process. The last REM period, or periods, may even eventually succeed in coming up with a successful way of solving serious dilemmas.

The emotional content of the dream varies directly with daytime emotionality. In young, normal individuals dream affect is most often neutral in tone. When dreams show evidence of conflict, this is usually linked to a troubling life situation. Normal individuals undergoing divorce showed distress in their dreams more often than those who had stable marital existences, according to a classic study. Eighty-six percent of the divorcing sample had threatening dreams, but such dreams occurred in only fifty-six percent of a married control sample. Anxiety appeared twice as often for those who were divorcing. Their last dream of the night was negative, whereas the last dreams of the happily married were mostly positive. One patient of mine, who married and divorced a number of times, described having frequent dreams during divorce episodes that the airplanes in which he was flying would crash.

A number of experiments have demonstrated significant correlation between the day's experience and dreams. In one experiment subjects wore red goggles the entire day for a period of five to eight days. Dream reports from this period were collected. Every subject had dreams with red or orange color and colored lights, and no blue or green images were found. This "goggle effect" ended quickly after their removal.

Patients with anorexia and bulimia show dream preoccupation with eating and drinking. They also tend to have Lilliputian dreams in which persons and objects are markedly reduced in size.

Other experiments showed that tests involving anagram tasks presented prior to bedtime resulted in different dream levels of conflict, depending upon whether the puzzle was solved or unsolved by bedtime; unsolved problems showed higher dream references. Action films which are shown prior to sleep induce stress and result in higher levels of dream anxiety than neutral, stress-free films.

Posttraumatic Stress Disorder Dreaming

Posttraumatic stress disorder is a condition caused by the experience of an unusual, life threatening circumstance. The victim is later plagued by involuntary daytime flashbacks which revive the original trauma. The trauma is also reproduced in the experience of nightmarish dreams, resulting in an intense insomnia typical of this disorder. The flashbacks have been seen as an attempt at belated mastery of the threat of the original trauma. A woman who had experienced the occupation of her country by the Nazis when she was a child during World War II, frequently had recurring dreams involving persecution and death threats from Nazis. A siren heard during the day was a sufficient stimulus to induce a flashback in which she relived a violent threatening episode from the Nazi occupation.

Sufferers from this disorder frequently resort to alcohol to numb themselves enough to fall asleep, or to reduce daytime anxiety. Use of alcohol in these circumstances is a two-edged sword, since the violent upsurge of anxiety dream ideation that follows the wearing off of the alcohol induced REM suppression, is extremely agitating and sleep disrupting.

Presleep Experience and Dreaming

A series of experiments attempted to show correlations between various stimuli presented during sleep, especially during REM periods, and their incorporation into dream scenarios. The dream representations of such actual stimuli as drops of water dripping on the forehead, the tickling of the nose and other parts of the face with feathers, as well as the ringing of bells, and similar manipulations, were studied. The results showed that the experimental stimuli did not appear in the dream; if they did, it was in nonessential ways that were not central to the dream narrative. The influence of presleep thinking on dream activity is striking, however, where problem solving is an important element in the dream. This is illustrated by the well-known report of the way the structure of the benzene ring was solved for Kekule in a dream when he had the dream image of six snakes in a circle nipping each others' tails. Another classic example is Elias Howe's solution of the problem of inventing a workable sewing machine needle when he had a dream of a spear with a hole in the head. In the arts, Coleridge, Robert Louis Stevenson, and Edgar Allan Poe all received inspirations for their creations from dreams.

There have also been investigations into whether the close correlation between REM sleep and penile erections has the associated effect of an increase in erotic dream content. The results have been largely negative. As a matter of fact, there is a low level of sexual content in dreams in general. Exceptions to this occur when anxiety levels are raised. In such cases, the manifest sexuality of dream content is increased. Exercise done before sleep seems to increase the possibility of sexual content, probably caused by an increase in arousal and the affiliation effect (described in chapter 16).

Dream Contents

Dreams have been studied for their content. A major study completed in 1950 analyzed the content of dreams in terms of the following opposing elements: characters in dreams; whether male or female; familiar or unfamiliar; aggression in dreams; friendliness; befriended or befriendor; sex; misfortune; settings and whether indoor or outdoor; and objects.

This study was repeated in the 1980s, and compared with the previous study to evaluate the effect of the major cultural changes that took place in the interval. The review showed a surprising stability of the nature of dream contents in the interim, despite certain significant changes. The previously noted differences between men and women on certain items had leveled out. Aggression and its manifestations in women, which had originally been much lower than men's, were more like those of men in the later study. In addition, there was more emphasis on thinking in the dreams of women, a supposedly more masculine quality. These changes were assumed to reflect the cultural effects of the sexual revolution.

Sleep Research and Dreams

It was found that about eighty-five percent of all dreams could be recalled by awakening subjects in the sleep laboratory when the EEG showed REM activity. At first it was thought that dreams took place only during REM. Later investigations showed, however, that dreaming also took place during NREM. The dreams in this phase of sleep, however, dealt with more mundane subjects which were not richly elaborated and stuck quite closely to the concerns of the subject's everyday world. Some investigators think that NREM dreams are really REM dreams which have lingered out of phase.

The techniques that were established to study dreams covered both dreams occurring in the home as well as those in the laboratory and have, through this wider scope, enabled investigators to study dreaming more systematically and scientifically.

Hypnagogic (occurring on going to sleep) and hypnopompic (occurring on waking) hallucinations are not restricted in their occurrence to narcolepsy but may arise in other circumstances, being REM dream variants of a special type. A culturally determined example of a hypnagogic hallucination, described to me by one of my patients, is the appearance of the "Boog" at sleep onset and waketimes. The patient stated that many of his friends and relatives living in the Carolinas had experienced this phenomenon, with sleep paralysis occurring in conjunction with a hypnagogic hallucination in which a terrifying figure is seen to be running around the bed and threatening the sleeper. Presumably the name derives from the idea of a bogeyman. A variant of this phenomenon occurs in Newfoundland. In this case the frightening figure is an old woman called "the Hag."

Whereas dream research psychologists focus on the phenomena which appear in the dream, other investigators have approached dreams from the opposite direction, focusing on the underlying physiological activity of the brain itself. The latter speculate that sensory and motor input from outside of the body is shut off during REM. Instead, spontaneous and random stimuli arising from the brainstem are believed to excite perceptual thinking and emotional organization when they reach the forebrain. It is speculated that the mind of the dreamer has a synthesizing function capable of matching up randomly activated neural systems with memory bank material. With such haphazard interconnectedness playing a large role, it cannot be expected that dreams would be logical—their bizarreness is implicit in the process. This theory is called the Activation-Synthesis Model of dreaming.

In the parasomnia called REM Behavior Disorder, the normal inhibition of motor activity that is typical of REM sleep is lifted, owing to either a psychiatric or medical disorder. The individuals who suffer from this sleep problem are thus able to physically act out their dreams since their motor function is not paralyzed during REM. These acted out dreams are frequently of a violent nature.

The dreams contain scenes of being attacked by animals or strangers. The emotional tone in the dreams is that of great fear with attempts at either fighting back or flight. The dreams are associated with defensively motivated, agitated, and violent behavior, which may have dangerous consequences for a bed partner as well as for the dreamer.

Laura Levin's husband died, leaving her with a house with a large mortgage which strapped her financially, creating severe stress in her life. This stress plus the grief over her husband's death caused her to develop a major depression. Her sleep at this time began to be characterized by episodes of rising from bed and going to the door of her bedroom, where she would usually abruptly awaken. She had dreams periodically, during this course of events, of being in a room which was totally enclosed, and when she would go to the door, it couldn't be opened, or would actually be a part of the wall itself, therefore frustrating her efforts to escape. The sleepwalking and the dreams clearly show her attempt to elude the mortgage stress, but also demonstrate her feeling of being trapped within that house and situation. With psychological and pharmacological treatment the REM behavior disorder parasomnia and frustration based dreaming ceased.

The extreme behaviors evidenced in REM behavior disorder dreams are atypical of the patient's normal personality. The change in ordinary dreaming content—to agitated themes of a nightmarish, violent, and repetitive nature—seen in REM behavior disorder dreaming, is typically sudden. REM behavior disorder most frequently occurs in the older population, with premonitory aspects of the illness present in these individuals in earlier age periods. Specific pharmacologic treatments, which are extremely effective, exist for this condition.

Nightmares

Nightmares are a special type of dream. They occur mostly in the second half of sleep, during a long REM period of twenty to thirty minutes. The dream action is accompanied by a feeling of terror, with the dreamer being chased, threatened, hurt, or killed. The usual escape is through waking. Screaming in the dream is frequent, although in reality it is seldom out loud. One theory assumes that nightmares are the result of oxygen deprivation in the brain.

Studies of sleep apnea, where there is oxygen deprivation when breathing periodically stops, show, however, that nightmares are absent at these times.

The term nightmare derives from the Old English word "mare," meaning demon. Nightmares occur at any age. Children between the ages of three and five have enough nightmares to cause their parents concern. Nightmares diminish with age. College undergraduates who were studied, reported a frequency of approximately ten a year, whereas the average annual number in the older age groups is about three. Older persons, especially those with obstructive apnea, however, report great concern about nightmares. For all of us, having current problems increases their frequency. A small group have them regularly, often more than once a week. Nightmares express feelings of helplessness on the part of the dreamer. Nightmares are founded in reality situations. They are not alien and abstract but quite personal, concrete, and intensely relevant to the dreamer. Heart rates and breathing rates increase during nightmares, as might be expected. Nightmares can even occur during napping, particularly when the nap lasts an hour or longer.

The small group of people who have a long history of nightmares dating back to childhood, manifest special personality characteristics. Studies show that although they are not especially neurotic, anxious, or hostile in their daily lives, they report feeling somewhat different from the rest of the population from childhood on. In their personalities, they are the opposite of the controlled, rigid, down-to-earth types. Nightmare-prone persons are pictured as open, trusting, and creative, and are described by personality theorists as having "thin ego boundaries." This term means they have difficulty in separating fantasy from reality, and during the day they in fact may often drift off into daydreams.

Their sense of self-identity is rather unclear to them, and in dreams they frequently can abruptly assume another identity, even one of a lower-order being. They are emotionally thin skinned and highly empathic—sensitive to the feelings of others. They have excellent past memories which reach all the way back to their earliest years. They are extremely intuitive. Their openness makes them vulnerable, not only to the anxieties manifested in their nightmares, but also in terms of their real-life interpersonal relationships.

Sudden increases of nightmarish dreams that are accompanied with severe insomnia can be the prelude to an episode of major mental problems.

Other Dream Types

Psychiatric states are highly correlated with dream scenarios. Dreaming is decreased in severe depressions and, when dreams occur, they become shorter and more unpleasant, although they don't have the full character of a true nightmare. Dreaming becomes longer in length and more typical in structure, as well as brighter in illumination, as recovery from a depression proceeds.

An increase in dreaming, with a high content of vivid dreams about body changes, accompanies pregnancy and, in some cases, may be the first sign of conception even though a woman may not realize she is pregnant. People suffering from febrile illnesses or painful conditions also report more dreaming, probably because their symptoms cause more awakenings, and as a result, more recall. Certain drugs, among them beta blockers and L-Dopa, either cause nightmares or increase their frequency. Rapid withdrawal from antidepressants and excessive use of BDZs may have similar effects.

Lucid Dreaming

In the type of dream known as Lucid Dreaming, dreamers become aware they are dreaming and are able to introduce elements of volitional control into the dream. If we dream of flying, for example, this control may take the form of becoming the pilot, controlling the flight of the body in various directions, swooping up and down, or even coming in for landings. Lucid dreams are usually pleasurable in nature. The ability to be conscious of dreaming and to exercise control over it, is in marked contrast to the usual passivity that characterizes dreams. Lucid dreaming is an REM phenomenon, but a rare one; only about five percent of the population have regular lucid dream phenomena. Lucid dreams are not caused by microawakenings during sleep. They are far removed from awakening, since they occur in a deep REM state.

Various strategies have been attempted to increase lucid dream frequency, including posthypnotic suggestion, special training, and sensory stimulation during REM sleep periods. Special goggles have been utilized. Red lights are triggered when REM sleep occurs, and arouse the dreamer enough to be marginally conscious while dreaming. Subjects are instructed before sleep to signal with wrist or eye movements when dreaming, indicating lucidity. Some subjects are found to be remarkably sensitive, and are able to signal awareness through most REM dream episodes.

Lucid dreams are more likely to occur in later REM periods of the night. Arousal signs during lucid sleep are minimal. Although presleep hypnotic suggestion helps induce lucid dreaming, suggestibility, and other personality characteristics that are usually associated with hypnotizability, are not significantly present in the personality structure of the lucid dreamer. Indeed, there have been no consistent features of personality found that are able to predict which person will be a lucid dreamer.

Lucid dreaming is under intense investigation, since it has potential for important clinical applications. The treatment of nightmares and phobias, the resolution of emotional conflicts, and the enhancement of creativity are among the goals of lucid dream research.

The Senoi culture in Malaysia used lucid dreaming to diminish fears of enemies. Dreams of the previous night were avidly discussed among these people. Under the tutelage of tribal leaders, who acted as primitive psychotherapists, tribal members were trained from childhood to attain control over their dream thinking and even to induce dreams. Through the use of premeditated programmed dreaming, they were able to rid themselves of many kinds of fears and phobias. As a result, social conflict among these people was virtually eliminated. They were also able to dream of defeating their enemies. The sense of security achieved through the dream victories helped to make actual battle with other tribes unnecessary, since the Senoi seemed magically potent and overwhelming. They lived in peace.

Therapeutic Use of Dreams

The applied use of dreams has an ancient lineage. In Delphi, Greece, temples devoted to dream incubation were combined with oracular interpretation to cure dreamers of illness, or guide them in handling life's problems. Narcosynthesis is a modern variation of these techniques. This latter method was particularly popular during and after World War II, when it was enlisted to deal with the posttraumatic stress disorders of soldiers and veterans, helping to resolve their anxiety-laden experiences of flashbacks and night-mares. In this technique, the subject is brought to a state of twilight sleep through intravenous barbiturate injection. While in this state the subject is induced, through persuasion and suggestion, to relive the traumatic episode, in this way overcoming the symptoms of the stress disorder.

I employed this technique with a young married woman who suffered from dissociated psychic states, known as fugue episodes. These occurred as part of her multiple personality disorder. Such patients, in ordinary life, do not recall the episodes occurring in their other personalities. Using narcosynthesis, I was able to get her to re-experience a typical fugue episode by putting her into a quasisleep state. While in this state of mind, she was able to recall and describe the experiences taking place in a fugue in which she took a nighttime trip by ferry from Long Island to Connecticut. In her twilight state she described coming into port in Connecticut. She saw the dock and shore as a fairyland, with magical, lanternlike lights shining in the dark. The scene was experienced in an uplifted spirit of joy. The world opened up to her with a sense of childlike wonderment by slipping into an altered state during her ferry ride, demonstrating how tenaciously she clung to the re-enacted world of her childlike views.

Interpretation of Dreams

The interpretations of dream thinking vary with the particular school of dream theory in their concepts of motivations, dyna-misms, and the nature of humans. In the phenomenological ap-proach, which I use in understanding dream material, the dreamer is seen to exist in as real a world during the dream as during the day. Dreams reflect the dreamer's real relationships and are ex-pressions of the dreamer's being. Ghosts are experienced as real ghosts to the dreamer, and animals are real animals from this point of view. Dream objects and relationships do not have to be reduced to other things by symbolization and distortion.

A patient who dreams of seeing the dictator Mussolini is de-

scribing her feelings of being in a real relationship with a real dictator, her mother in the day world in this case. A dream of seeing
a water wheel shows the dreamer's existence as going round and
round in circles. A psychologically detached man's dream of seeing
the Einsteinian equation $E = MC^2$, shows the abstract nature of
this dreamer's existence. Just as the positions assumed by the
dreamer in sleep show the positions assumed by the dreamer in
waking life, so do dreams show the attunements of the individual's
existence to the real world he or she inhabits. In a life attuned to
hunger, dreams reveal eatable things and scenes of dining.

The major distinction between dream life and waking life is that
when the dreamer wakes, historical reality, with day to day continuity, is confronted. This does not exist in dreamworld events,
where the usual constraints of time and space are of a different
order than daytime logic.

Recurrent Dreams

Recurring dreams occur frequently in posttraumatic stress disorder. They also occur with nightmares. A traumatic event at a young
age may, in some cases, be followed by reliving the event in the
form of a repetitive nightmare that recurs throughout life; the
script of the nightmare may change, but the essential theme of
the trauma remains the same. The context chosen will explicate
the maturing individual's conflict-laden experiences in terms of the
story line and the scenario of the dream.

For example, one of my patients was traumatized as a child when
she saw the movie version of S. S. Van Dine's classic mystery novel,
The Cat and the Canary. In the book, and in the film made from
it, visitors to a spooky old castle were systematically murdered night
after night. Each victim stood against a wall on which a picture
hung. When the person was alone, the picture behind them was
moved to one side revealing a catlike creature wearing a mask and
a black costume. This creature extended its arms and clawed hands,
and choked the unfortunate prey to death. My patient remembered
cowering when seeing the film, especially in scenes where a catlike
black appendage appeared through the hole in the wall.

In later life she had frequent nightmares recalling this particular
set of images. This turned into a plaguing insomnia. Not only did
this material appear in her dreams but even extended into her

daytime life. She suffered from phobias and was always frightened of the possibility of intruders breaking into her apartment. She kept her doors and windows tightly locked.

One day when seated at an outdoor cafe a cat rubbed itself against her leg. This catalytic event led to a severe cat phobia so that even seeing the picture of a cat gave her an immediate anxiety reaction. Cat nightmares increased, resulting in the severe disturbances of sleep and resultant fatigue during the day.

The information she presented during her treatment revealed that the cause of her cat phobia and insomnia lay not only in the movie of *The Cat and the Canary*, but extended to more significant causal circumstances. Her parents' marriage was conflicted and her father was a distant and threatening figure. She spent much time at her maternal grandparents' home and as a child often slept with her kindly grandfather. She reported noticing that while he was asleep in bed with her his darkened penis would often protrude from his pajamas, probably in REM erection. She was both stimulated and frightened by the sight. This material was later replaced by the memory of the film's image of a catlike black appendage. The actual outbreak of the cat phobia occurred at the time of a growing emotional attachment to a charismatic male employer. What she experienced as a child and reexperienced with a cat unexpectedly rubbing itself against her chair and leg, was the emergence and pressure of her own carnal existence, which she, for various reasons felt would overwhelm her. The function of the phobia and nightmares was to keep this material and its implications at a distance.

Over the course of my psychotherapeutic work I've noticed that women tend to identify with cats in dreams, whereas men more frequently identify with dogs. Paralleling this is the frequency with which women have cat phobias and men dog phobias.

* * *

Our nighttime dreaming frequently ends traumatically. The male patient who was married and divorced many times, flies often in real life as well as in his dreams. In his dreams, as noted, he often crashes. Similarly, his real existence has many crashes primarily of a romantic nature. In the dream crises, planes are smashed yet he emerges unscathed and walks away. He remarked on the fact that despite all these traumatic events no blood is seen. The ability to eliminate blood, the vital essence of life, showed that the dreamer perceived that it was really dream fear he experienced, and not life.

A special instance of this ability to perceive such important differences is shown by the phenomenon of dreams within dreams, in which the dreamer dreams of having a dream, adding a detaching layer of distance to involvement in the dream events.

Chapter 19

Uncoverings

New Findings

We have seen an enormous growth in sleep research since the discovery of REM sleep in 1953. The prime catalyst of this development has been technological in nature. The collection of data in an objective, standardized way has been a major achievement of polysomnography and other laboratory procedures. A recent advance has been an increased emphasis on clinical and office practices dealing with the treatment of the insomnias. A particularly fruitful result of this new direction has been the augmented availability of clinical observations, leading to the uncovering of interesting and valuable insights concerning both sleep and insomnia.

This chapter presents previously unknown phenomena and experiences which I have seen revealed in my own clinical work. This material has not appeared in the literature as far as I have been able to ascertain.

The Set Point Theory of Insomnia

In the Set Point theory of weight, the body clings to a fixed level of weight, resisting up or down variations caused by overeating or dieting. The theory assumes that the body deals with processes of rapid physiological change like a ship's governor, holding its balance as long as possible at a set position before yielding to the pressure of change. The body's tendency to resist change is called Homeostasis. Homeostasis seems to work the same way in insomnia as in weight, each of us having a preference for a given amount of sleep.

I've been struck by a regularly occurring pattern. The observation applies the set point concept to the process of sleep loss. When sleep is lost in chronic insomnia, it takes place in a stepwise manner; varying in a continuum, with the body establishing a series of periodic equilibrium (set) points during ongoing episodes of sleep loss. Changes are gradually modulated along this series of nodal points rather than in random fluctuations. In this way, control against instability is maintained. This stepwise pattern of sleep loss is clearly seen when we keep logs of average losses on a weekly basis.

Recovery from insomnia and return to normal sleep amounts appears to operate somewhat differently than the loss pattern, occurring much more rapidly and without the inclination to rally around nodal points.

This leads to the conclusion that in sleep loss the body fights a defensive rearguard action, with only gradual yielding of sleep time. As the trend toward loss continues, various lines of defense against further attrition are called into play until there is a rally. At this point, the amount of sleep lost is maintained for a period. The loss seems to be that amount of sleeplessness which can be tolerated by the individual's physiology at that particular time; it is held at this quantum until the forces interfering with sleep can no longer be withstood. The sleep loss level now falls to a new, lower rallying point. This pattern seems to hold across the board for the insomnia cases which I have seen. With recovery from insomnia (regardless of the factors that interfered with sleep, and whatever the individual defenses used to deal with the sleep loss) the process of relief appears to rebound in an all-or-nothing way, with normal sleep levels being regained as rapidly as possible.

Sleep and the Masking Phenomenon

Have you ever been in the shower and imagined hearing the phone ring? This is an example of the Masking Phenomenon. It also occurs in connection with sleep.

The masking phenomenon is a common occurrence. An environment loses its familiar features for us as a result of the masking, which obliterates our cuing and organizing abilities. We are relatively disorganized and under stress to make sense of the new environment until reorientation sets in.

The transition to sleep is often associated with anxiety. Factors such as assuming the horizontal position, the loss of day world structure during the sleep phase, the passivity of sleep with loss of the sense of control, and the opening up to the unknown in terms of dream experience, all foster a regressive state that can be fraught with anxiety for some. This regressive state may also be brought about by other events, such as sensory deprivation, the use of drugs, highly charged emotional stimuli, or during a phase of heightened creativity. In the examples to be described, the individual reorganizes the environment to offset the masking. The way the situation is reorganized becomes a sort of inkblot test, where the person projects his or her own organizing pattern. The pattern that is projected is typically that of a preoccupying unresolved conflict, if the situation is emotionally charged, as demonstrated in the following cases.

John Chubb, a young man, experienced difficulty falling asleep during warm weather because of the need to use an air conditioner at this time of year. The hum of the air conditioner blocked out the familiar sounds of his urban environment and allowed the following masking phenomenon to occur. As he was falling asleep with the air conditioner droning, he would suddenly imagine hearing his father's voice speaking in a loud and disturbed manner.

The origin of this hypnagogic hallucination at sleep onset was his experiences with sleep as a child. His father, who suffered from a mental disorder that recurred periodically, would at these times awaken the sleeping household with episodes of ranting and excitable talk caused by his mental disturbance. This experience left a marked imprint on this young man, creating great anxiety in him. He had a particular fear of inheriting a mental problem as a consequence of his identification with his father, in effect, the frightening possibility of "like father, like son."

There were other ramifications in this case. The young man was quite obsessive-compulsive and, like others having this personality trait, had a great need to be forever in control. During his developing years his bedroom was next door to his parents' room. Their sexual activity, rather than being discreet, ran in the opposite direction; the love sounds they made were clearly heard in the son's adjacent bedroom, often preventing him from falling asleep, or even awakening him from deep sleep. These eruptions proved so disturbing to him that he had to bang on the wall to get them to reduce the sound volume of their vocal and physical sexual expressions. This stark experience was of importance in his case. He heard his father's disturbed ranting overtly in the masking phenomenon. Behind this behavior lay his fear of arousal. The original bedroom episodes were, despite their disruptive quality, extremely exciting to him. A fear of loss of control over his emotions was kindled by the stimulating associations to the air conditioner noise. It was no surprise to find that he suffered from sexual difficulties that were also caused by fear of loss of control. The regressive correlation of the themes of sleep and sex resulted in an interference with his ability to give up control, relax, and fall asleep at night when the air conditioner was on.

Analogous illustrations of the masking phenomenon are the occurrence of bogeyman fears in children and sundowning in the elderly, who both need a night-light left on to reassure themselves against the regressive fears which arise in unstructured darkness. Another example is the case I have already described of the pregnant woman left on a table in a laboratory, who later, in the last trimester of her pregnancy, developed a hallucination of awakening from sleep thinking she was hearing a phone ringing.

Sounds that are regular and result in a smooth, unstructured perception-masking ambiance, seem very apt to result in hearing nonexistent noises. This happens frequently with showers. The running water creates a continuous thrumming which blankets out other sounds and creates a masking effect. In one instance, a woman patient would routinely experience hearing her husband cry out in pain whenever she showered before going to sleep. In a panic she would leap out of the shower and run dripping into the bedroom to discover her husband lying peacefully in bed. The masking phenomenon of the shower caused her to hallucinate the sound of his voice.

The basis of her insecurity was the fact that her husband had recently suffered a heart attack. As a consequence, she had developed a hypervigilance to protect him. Her ability to hear a possible cry for help was covered up by the masking noise of the shower, causing the emergence of her anxiety and her panicky run to his aid. Similarly, a young boy complained that he could always hear his mother scolding and yelling at him whenever he took a shower or was in any situation where fans or air conditioners were running.

An interesting parallel to this masking shower phenomenon occurred during the time when Alfred Hitchcock's thriller *Psycho* was first showing in movie theaters. In this classic film, a young woman checked into a motel on a stormy night and prepared for bed. She was murdered in the shower with the camera focusing on horrifying camera shots of blood trickling down to the shower floor. The film left such an indelible imprint of terror that I've had a number of patients tell me that the development of their own masking phenomena was stimulated by seeing it.

For example, one young man related that after seeing the film he always left the bathroom door open when he was taking a shower. If he did not do this, he would inevitably feel that an intruder had entered his apartment without his being able to hear, and that the intruder was going to assault him in the shower.

In another case, a female patient would always rush, awash and in fright, from her prebed shower on the assumption that during the blackout of outside sound when she was under the tap, an intruder had entered into her apartment. She would dash into the living room and there in a large chair with its back to her, she would think that she could perceive someone sitting in the dark. This false perception scared her out of her wits. Her fears were groundless, of course, and were the result of very special, personal historical circumstances. As in the young man's case, her bedtime shower masking experiences were also caused by seeing *Psycho*.

The masking phenomenon is not infrequent and should be considered in applicable histories when dealing with sleep onset or sleep maintenance insomnia.

Sleep and the Isakower Phenomenon

The Isakower Phenomenon, named after its discoverer, is another example of a regressive, hypnagogic condition. Individuals feel that there is a white mass floating above their heads in this experience, and that their faces, especially the mouth parts, are enormously enlarged. This enlargement mainly involves the tongue, the lips, and the jaw. In addition, a special crinkly sensation of the skin is experienced in the upper parts of the body, the shoulders, the upper arms, or the cheeks. It was felt that the phenomenon was the expression of a regression to an "oral stage fixation," caused by the same factors which we have described in the masking phenomenon.

In my experiences with insomnia patients, I have occasionally seen cases in which the Isakower phenomenon is associated with difficulties in falling asleep at sleep onset or in awakenings during the night. As noted, most patients who experience the phenomenon describe abnormal feelings of enlargement of the mouth or adjacent areas. The vague cloud was interpreted as representing the person's recall of the breast of the mother and her reassuring presence in the nursing situation of infancy. In the following case the hallucinatory phenomena consisted not of oral or perioral details but of the patient's feeling that his hands were enlarged. It was thought that hand involvement also related to nursing, since infants often touch the mother's breast in the suckling process. There was in this case, moreover, a definite perception of a white cloud mass, putting the experience clearly within the orbit of the Isakower phenomenon.

The patient was in his thirties and involved in a stressful separation and divorce. Often he would awaken during the night and examine his hands, experiencing the feeling that they had suddenly grown and were enormous. These experiences were of recent origin and seemed clearly associated with his marital stress. In his history, though, he was able to recall that he had first experienced an episode of a similar nature during puberty, roughly around the age of thirteen.

I could not elicit any significant information about his life situation at that time, and only noted the coincidence with puberty. I speculated that this phenomenon represented some guilt or anxiety about masturbation at that age, since the experience focused on his hands. The patient demonstrated strong compulsive trends in his personality. He was extremely precise about time and set two alarm clocks to be sure to awaken in the morning. He usually anticipated the first of these clocks as he would routinely awaken four minutes prior to its going off and never had to rely on the backup alarm. Focal psychotherapy as well as appropriate behavior therapy succeeded in reducing the episodes of the insomnia and the associated Isakower phenomenon. In his nighttime anxiety he was trying to overcome the trauma of separation from his spouse by the regressive compensatory recapture of the security image of the mother.

Compulsive Urination Insomnia

A frequent event, which I call Compulsive Urination Insomnia, interferes with falling asleep and is also associated with sleep maintenance problems. It is quite remarkable how many people experience this problem and yet how infrequently they spontaneously bring the topic up for discussion when seen in a standard medical consultation. As I have described in my workup, I routinely ask questions about the possibility of compulsive urination during my initial interview with an insomnia patient. The overlooking, or covering up, by patients of repeated bouts of compulsive urination at night is owing, perhaps, to the connection of this material with the shameful area of excretion and toilet training. Feelings of sensitivity about apparent loss of control in this sector may also play a role. I've found it fruitful in all cases of insomnia, especially in those individuals with a strong compulsive component to their personality, to inquire about such episodes.

Most of us regularly and ritually void our urine at bedtime and perhaps if we awaken during the course of the night. This midcourse procedure is especially marked in older males with prostatic enlargement and, to a lesser extent, in women who have weakening of the urethral sphincter.

Compulsive urination is quite different from these standard situations. As a cause of sleep disturbance, it occurs much more frequently in the younger age groups and can affect women as often as men. When urinating is not associated with compulsivity, the individual usually is satisfied with the single voiding episode and goes back to bed and to sleep. In compulsive urination the psychological dynamics interfere with this process.

In voiding there is always a small amount of residual urine left in the bladder. Some compulsive individuals, in order to insure being able to sleep without being awakened by further stimulation from the slight feeling of pressure in the bladder from the residual urine, get out of bed and go to the bathroom again. They usually manage to squeeze out the small amount of urine that was left in the bladder or that was produced subsequent to the previous void-

ing. To increase the sense of security that results, they try to eliminate all such bladder sensations completely by voiding again and
again. This back and forth activity can become ritualized so that
the repeated urinations take on the force of a compulsive practice.
I have had patients tell me that the repeated voidings can take
place as many as thirty or forty times in a prebed period or when
awakened during the night and trying to get back to sleep.

In many cases the ritual has become so extensive that it has even
penetrated daytime behavior, requiring frequent reassuring trips
to the bathroom during work, for example. This daytime urinary
frequency symptom is familiar to urologists, but their patients seem
to avoid talking about any association with insomnia. It appears to
be more acceptable to present this problem as a daytime symptom
about which organic origins can be assumed and searched for. In
the case of nighttime compulsive urination, it is clearer that psychogenic factors are often in operation; this tends to create re-
pression of the correlation in presenting the history.

As mentioned, frequency of urination is common among older
males because of prostatic enlargement. Even here, however, because of a linkage with tendencies to compulsiveness, the component of magic ritual may take hold and add to the increase in
sleep difficulties. Older women who have difficulty with sphincter
control and suffer from involuntary voiding are also vulnerable to
the development of compulsive urination insomnia. Patients tell
me that when they plan extended automobile journeys they factor
in strategic stops at gas stations and other points to ensure themselves of having the opportunity to engage in the necessary voiding ritual.

In one case, a patient was prevented from taking advantage of
the opportunity to travel because of this problem. He was afraid
to visit friends and relatives out of town since he was fearful of
calling attention to his difficulties by his repeated trips to the bathroom and toilet flushings at night. This caused an insomnia if he
dared to undertake a visit. His shame was so great that even traveling to locations where no one knew him, but where his pattern
might be observed or heard, made such journeys taboo. His problem was overcome by the simple suggestion that he keep a plastic
urinal by his bed when visiting or traveling, to prevent his compulsive voiding from being noticed. The further resolution of the
causes of his insomnia and the lessening of his psychological need

for the ritual was of great help in his case; enabling him to redis-cover the joy of travel and the freedom of social motion.

The Lightness and Darkness of Being in Dreams

Dream analysis has become quite sophisticated. Contemporary theories of dream interpretation and the use of dream content analysis, as well as the research in sleep physiology, have contrib-uted to this. In my own work with sleep patients I have noticed another parameter involved in reports of dreams that I find signif-icant for clinical work, and which has proven extremely useful to me in terms of evaluating a patient's clinical standing. This is the occurrence of the elements of light or dark in dream reports. I have found that reports of a well-lit or a more darkened environ-ment occurring in a dream is an extremely sensitive indicator of the mood of the dreamer, with a strong parallel between these qualities and the emotion the dreamer is experiencing in life.

When the dream takes place in an environment of darkness, or lowered light intensity, this event seems to be correlated with the experience of depression or a lowered mood in the dreamer's life. On the other hand, the experience of bright light in the dream environment shows optimism, buoyancy, and an overall mood el-evation. In following the dreams of a depressed person it is inter-esting to note that as the patient's mood lifts the incidence of re-ported bright light increases.

The indexing of the degree of light or darkness in dreams can be added to other useful signs in evaluating whether a treated pa-tient is recovering from depression. It can even help in making a diagnosis of whether a depression is truly present in unclear cases. As patients recover from a depression there is an increased ten-dency to report the existence of colors in dreams, and the presence of progressively warmer colors tends to correlate with recovery from the depressed state.

It is of interest that, as in the case of speech in dreams, there is no definition of the source of light, whether sun or moon, electric light, or otherwise. Light, like sound, seems to just be there.

Sleep Positions and Psychopathology

My work on sleep positions showed the strong correlations that exist between sleep positions and psychological structure. One of my psychiatric colleagues was intrigued by this observation and applied the information to inpatients on the hospital wards that were under his supervision. Patients in the hospital are routinely checked every hour during the night by nursing personnel and their condition is charted in the case record. My colleague trained his ward staff to chart the sleep positions of patients under his care according to my classification system. In this way, over a period of time, he amassed a record of 2,200 separate observations of the individual sleep positions of his psychiatric patients.

In analyzing results with him, we made the following observations. Most patients suffering from a major depressive episode were recorded as assuming a full fetal sleep position for most of the night during their hospital stay. This sleep position was uniform in those patients suffering from major depressions, regardless of the normal basic personality of the patients and their usual preferred sleep positions.

In addition to the close relationship between major depression and the assumption of the full fetal sleep position in this case material, another strong psychopathological correlation was noticed in paranoid males. I had already noted this connection in my own clinical work with patients in my private psychiatric practice. In both situations, during outbreaks of psychiatric stress these patients would change their sleep position from whatever it was normally to the royal sleep position, on their backs. This seemed paradoxical, since the psychologically decompensating individual, faced with stress and threat, might have been expected to protect himself by assuming either a full fetal position or sleeping prone to decrease vulnerability of his vital organs during sleep.

I reason that this seemingly paradoxical preference for the royal position in these cases can be understood in terms of the underlying conflict of the male paranoid patient. This conflict centers around anal concerns and the conflicted desire for, and fear of, anal penetration. It follows, therefore, that when they consider themselves highly vulnerable, as in a stressful or psychiatric conflict situation, they would guard themselves in their sleep by assuming the royal position, that is, in vulgar parlance, "cover their ass." That they thereby make themselves more vulnerable in terms of the exposure of their vital centers, such as heart, genital, and digestive systems, is secondary to them in terms of their psychological defense needs. As in major depressions, it was again impressive to note that as soon as their psychological condition improved, they immediately resumed their normal preferred sleep positions.

The extreme sensitivity of sleep positions as a psychological marker was shown by the rapidity with which sleep positions in patients changed with the beginning of clinical improvement. I have previously mentioned this sensitivity and how sleep positions are able to show subtle variations in a person's emotional status. When, through treatment, patients began to recover, or when their situations deteriorated, sleep position changes often immediately preceded the clinical observation of a change.

A case report that presented some puzzling aspects was included in the material which my colleague collated. The patient, a woman who normally slept in the royal position, suffered such a severe depression that she required hospitalization. Her preferred sleep position during the depression was not the anticipated full-fetal, but a semi-fetal one, on her side with both legs extended, one precisely on top of the other. Such a position shows a high degree of compliance as well as an inability to relax even in sleep. In studying her history we found she had been a preferred child; her personality was that of a dependent clinging type. In her late adolescence she had been an unfortunate Jewish victim of the Holocaust and was subjected to years of internment in a Nazi concentration camp.

I believe it was this distorting experience of severe stress, where the patient's survival depended upon complete compliance, and where she was under continual harrowing threat psychologically and physically—compounded by the enforced mass side-by-side sleeping situation within the barracks—that resulted in the evocation of her hospital sleep position. This position was determined by the extreme circumstance surrounding her later depressive illness which reactivated the period of earlier threat and stress. In this regression, she returned to the earlier sleep position which she associated with her ability to endure and survive under the life-threatening concentration camp conditions. As soon as she had responded to medication and treatment, from one night to the next, she resumed her normal royal sleep position and gave up the one assumed in her depression.

Lazybones

Approximately a decade ago I treated a woman suffering from a depression caused by a massive physical trauma. She was struck by a car, and suffered a concussion, right knee and pelvis fractures, and a massive compound fracture of her right lower leg. When I saw her she had been operated on by an orthopedist, who had reconstructed her shattered knee. The lower leg had been put in a cast. Her pelvic fracture had healed. Although the cast had been removed, the healing of her lower leg had dragged on for many months, well beyond the usual healing period. She was severely depressed when I first saw her, and I started her on moderately high dosages of a tricyclic antidepressant. Within a number of weeks she was responding favorably to the antidepressant, and had emerged from her profound dysphoria. At this point she returned to her orthopedist for a checkup and, astonishingly, the fracture seemed to have suddenly healed.

The change seemed so remarkable that my curiosity was piqued and I checked the literature on possible connections between antidepressant use and bone healing. My review turned up a few notes and one major article on the topic. The implications of the citations, which at that time were all about ten years old, was that in some manner antidepressants stimulated activity of osteoblasts, the bone-forming cells of the body. I contacted some pharmaceutical houses that manufacture antidepressants for further information, but did not discover anything more on this topic. I left the issue in limbo at this point, but kept the clinical observation in mind until four years ago, when I was presented with a remarkably similar set of circumstances.

In this case, a male patient in his late forties was driving in a car which veered off the road and overturned, resulting in a fracture of the left collarbone and a compound fracture of the left lower leg. The orthopedic surgeon in this case handled the collarbone fracture with a shoulder sling, which brought the edges of the break into approximation, and surgically corrected the leg fracture by a bone transplant. The wound over the fracture was corrected by plastic surgery and the leg was placed in a cast. I was called into the case to deal with the patient's generalized anxiety and his resultant intense insomnia. I treated the insomnia with a moderate dosage level of sedating tricyclic antidepressant. Bearing in mind my previous experience with antidepressants and bone healing, I waited to see the effects in this particular case.

Until this point, the collarbone fracture did not seem to be heal-ing. The edges were wide apart and there was a wedge shaped chip of bone between the fracture ends. It seemed to me that the sur-geon, according to his reported remarks, was preparing the patient for a false joint as a possible outcome of this fracture. In examining the very next set of X rays, the orthopedist seemed puzzled and asked for repeat X rays of the fracture, apparently not believing what he saw. The collarbone had healed beautifully in the interim between visits. The patient continued the mild use of the antide-pressant for sleep purposes.

About six or seven months later the patient was making progress with his recovery from the leg fracture and was starting to put weight on the leg. The surgeon, though, was discouraged with the rate of healing and, at this point, presented the patient with two options; a new operation with further use of bone transplants to splint the fracture, or ultraconservative treatment with all weight off the leg. The patient chose the conservative program, although this would increase the length of his rehabilitation. He was also depressed about the possibility that he might eventually need fur-ther surgery with no guarantees. To add to his burdens, at this point his business underwent a severe crisis, putting him under extreme economic duress. The patient's depression and insomnia returned in ominous fashion.

I decided on recourse to full strength antidepressants in light of these developments. After some time, with the aid of the antide-pressant and intensive psychotherapy, the patient's mood lifted. This was aided by a turn for the better in his business. It was at this juncture that the periodic followups on his leg began to show increasingly better results in terms of the healing process. Today the patient walks on both legs, has given up the use of crutches and cane, and the leg seems well on its way to normal status.

I view this case as being quasiexperimental. The low dosage may have played a role in the sharp turnaround in the healing of the collarbone fracture, with the very close correlation to the intro-duction of the use of the low dose antidepressant. In the case of the leg fracture, the full-strength antidepressant may also have had beneficial effects on the eventual ability to dispense with a further surgical procedure to correct the fracture, and the ability to finally promote healing.

Tricyclic antidepressants have had many uses in medicine in addition to the purely psychiatric one of treating depressions. As noted, the literature hints they may have some effectiveness in promoting bone growth. If this is proved to be so, then they could be of value in other cases of need for higher bone growth activity, as in the major medical affliction of osteoporosis, a condition of brittle bones associated with advancing age, especially in women. The evidence in my two cases seems to point to this possibility.

Conditioned SAD

Anniversary reactions are recurrences of an original emotional trauma on the date in later years on which the original event happened.

In SAD, depressions occur either at the beginning of winter or summer.

When a parent suffers a recurring seasonal depression, children will experience repetitive losses of the parent's emotional presence. These children become vulnerable to experiences of depression at the seasonal time when the parent began to show signs of SAD. As a result, the children may become conditioned to periodic bouts of depression at the critical season. Even as independent adults they may suffer an anniversary reaction depression in winter or summer, although they themselves do not carry the intrinsic tendency to SAD.

Chapter 20

Sleep Fitness

Over the past two decades, the health and fitness concerns that once motivated the lives of a relative few have etched themselves into the general consciousness of our time. Jogging, aerobic exercises, concern for cholesterol levels, calorie intake, and nutrition across the board have become the bywords of millions. Yet the importance of the relationship of good sleep to total fitness has been largely overlooked. Although the majority of us take sleep for granted and are oblivious to the implications of sleep to the total fitness picture, the insomniac has no such misconceptions. Those suffering from continuing sleeplessness are only too aware now that poor sleep adversely affects daytime functions.

The evidence that sixty-nine plane accidents from 1983 to 1986 were linked to pilot fatigue, and that seventy billion dollars are lost annually by industry because of sleep difficulties of employees, underscores the importance of sleep to healthful functioning. An unexplained chilling statistic showed that sleepers who slept less than four hours or more than ten hours per day had significantly higher mortality rates.

On a purely physical level, athletes understand the relationship between good sleep and fitness. Professional athletes sleep more than seven and a half hours on the average and usually get nine hours of sleep per night during their playing season. Coaches know that there is a tendency for athletes to "go stale" if they break training rules and go to bed late. They enforce curfews for their athletes to maintain maximum states of fitness and insure peak performance.

It is not as simple as saying that exercise and good sleep go hand in hand, however. For the poor sleeper, exercise may make matters worse if it is pursued improperly. A leisurely stroll around the block before settling down for the hour of diminished activity called for by the rules of sleep hygiene can be beneficial. However, jogging a mile is likely to be so arousing as to hurt rather than help. Poor sleepers who get out of bed and do push-ups to tire themselves out are simply asking for more trouble. Exercise should be gradual and moderate for those not accustomed to a physically active life— too much and sleep will be disturbed. Any exercise program should be discussed with a physician for those with medical problems, of course.

In terms of diet, it is again not so much that good eating habits promote sleep, as that bad eating habits can be disruptive of sleep. It has been noted that this diet factor spans the generations: undernourished mothers have infants with disturbed sleep. Heavy or spicy foods consumed too close to lights-out time are likely to cause sleep problems, as has been noted here. Stimulants, like caffeine in coffee, can prove troublesome if they are ingested after late afternoon, whereas alcohol as a nightcap can have delayed effects that cause the sleeper to wake in the middle of the night.

Yet even people who use good sense about exercise and diet can encounter great difficulty sleeping. Sleep fitness is thus not just a result of other kinds of fitness but a separate category of fitness in and of itself. Good sleep has as profound an effect on daytime fitness as daytime activity has on sleep. It follows that our consciousness about the quality of sleep should be added to our consciousness about diet and exercise, and pursued with the same concern in a program of total fitness. The day world and the night world are markedly different spheres, but they are interdependent. Both daytime and nighttime events and activities need to be viewed as part of a unified ecosystem, each with its own role to play in our larger personal universe.

Consider, first, the role we play in the theater of the night. The bedroom serves as the setting for the bed that is the stage upon which we act out the drama of sleep. And, as we have seen, it is a large drama indeed, played out in three to four acts, each consisting of four stages of NREM sleep and a climactic REM stage. Extraordinary events take place. Skin, hair, and nail regeneration occur during sleep—it is quite accurately called beauty sleep. The clearing of the brain as an information processing system is accom-

plished during the night in preparation for the next day's mental work; many sleep researchers hold to the theory that this is the most important function of the REM phase of sleep, and a major reason that we require it. Others emphasize the production of both metabolic and sexual hormones during sleep, and the surge of temperature and adrenal hormone in the body at the end of the sleep period that energizes us for the coming day's activities.

The sleep drama encompasses numerous body movements as well as the paralysis of REM sleep. How remarkable it is that this paralysis should be accompanied by penile erections and clitoral engorgement, as well as the most intense dreams. There seems little doubt that there are many other complex and unknown events occurring during sleep that are only beginning to be discerned by sleep investigators. After all, most of the information in this book has been discovered and articulated only since the late 1960s.

It is one of the great paradoxes of sleep, however, that in order to experience this largely unconscious drama, we must relax into it. We lie down on the bed, the stage of the night, assuming a sleep position that is personally reassuring. Our sleep clothing—or lack of it if we choose nudity—must leave us feeling comfortable. The room must be cool enough to facilitate sleep entry. The lights have been dimmed or extinguished. Now we begin the withdrawal from a daytime world of action.

The abolition, as far as possible, of external stimuli is necessary to proceed into the world of sleep. If we sleep with a partner, the physical intimacy of bodily closeness to that person enhances security and adds a reassuring emotional resonance to our withdrawal from the day. The psychological emphasis is one of disengagement as the day's responsibilities are cast off along with its activities; even the more mature aspects of our relationship with the sleep partner are put aside and the bedroom attitude becomes more passive and more receptive.

That is what happens to good sleepers. But poor sleepers have a very different experience. They cannot let go of the day they have just lived through, or they may already be hurrying ahead to worry about tomorrow. In either case, they remain mentally aroused, and the body continues to reflect the adherent tension of daytime alertness.

This inability to let go can have many causes, as we have seen. For some individuals, a situation involving regression, diminished

perception, passivity, and intimacy may have anxiety-arousing con-
notations. This may result from the features of immobility and isolation in sleep that some people link with death. Compulsives, and
anxious people in general, are fearful of giving up vigilance against
threat, and regard limitation of movement as a lowering of their
defensive armamentarium. Depressives are more able to enter the
sleep world since it is the day world they fear, but toward daylight
they will awaken, filled with anxiety at once again having to deal
with a universe whose tone, to them, is doleful, demanding, and
criticizing.

Now it is another day. Poor sleepers tend to be more anxious,
depressed, worried, and more given to hypochondria during the
day than good sleepers. The debilitation caused by insomnia is
global, affecting nights, days, work, relaxation, sex, and family life.

Good sleepers, by contrast, are markedly more upbeat in daylight hours. They spend more time talking to other people, yet are
quite content to be alone, comfortable with themselves in either a
group situation or a solitary one. They are able to work efficiently.
They think more about their family and friends than poor sleepers
do. They have a much more active engagement in the day world,
both in terms of work and relationships.

Poor sleepers, focusing on their sleep problem, try to shut out
stimulation during the day in order to relax themselves for sleep at
night. The paradox that results from the contrasting styles of good
sleepers and poor sleepers is that the poor sleeper attempts to be
relaxed during the day, and then becomes aroused, active, and
unable to sleep at night. The good sleeper—the fit sleeper—is
active and alert during the day and relaxed and tranquil at night.

As the contrasting portraits of good sleepers and poor sleepers
make clear, the unique ways in which we live—which define us as
specific individuals—are encountered not only during the light of
day but also during the darkness of night. We do not hang up our
singular personalities in the closet when we come home at night.
We sleep as we live. All of us are inimitable persons by day, clearly
separate and identifiable in our uniqueness, but we also carry our
special personality hallmarks with us in our journey through the
night. The recognition that we are the same person, day or night,
is important to the successful treatment of insomnia, helping to
identify the essential forces creating the insomnia.

Until the very recent past, the success rate with chronic insomnia

was low—many patients suffered for twenty-five years or more. However, in the past dozen years, sleep science has made great forward strides. From the study of sleep positions to the technological breakthroughs, identification of new syndromes, and the discoveries pioneered by sleep investigators, our horizons are being continually broadened. New techniques for evaluating physiological events and brain activity during sleep, as well as clinical tactics for dealing with sleeplessness, have been enormously helpful in the treatment of insomnia patients. The added consideration of psychological and clinical parameters significantly enlarges the meaning and relevance of the physiological elements that are studied, and how these data should be interpreted and applied. In fact, a personality profile of an insomnia patient can be drawn that widens the scope of the physiological data yielded by polysomnography alone.

To begin we can add the standard psychiatric evaluation scale, which consists of a listing of the significant aspects of a psychiatric case. This includes the major presenting clinical syndrome, such as depression or posttraumatic stress disorder. Also included are the developmental and personality features, the medical conditions present, and the psychosocial stressors affecting the individual.

When we add to this list such parameters as the type of insomnia, the preferred sleep positions, and subjective factors—such as feelings about the quality of sleep—an even more detailed profile of the features of the insomnia can be realized. When the complementary psychological and clinical features are taken into consideration, the insomnia sufferer is seen as a person with a given life history and a unique personality who is afflicted with a particular pattern of sleeplessness.

As a result of viewing insomnia within this larger panorama—that combines clinical, laboratory, and psychological approaches—most of the cases of chronic sleeplessness that seemed intractable just a decade ago can be viewed in ways that are able to lead to more successful treatment. As we have seen, it is now possible for insomnia victims to be released from their purgatory. As the title of this book proclaims, it is now time to say *"Goodbye Insomnia: Hello Sleep."*

Appendix

Behavior Therapies for Insomnia

Stimulus Control Therapy

1. Establish a desired bedtime and waketime.
2. Plan a sedentary evening routine to begin thirty to sixty minutes before the desired bedtime.
3. Do not use the bed or bedroom for any activity other than sleep—except for sex.
4. Use regular presleep routines to associate with bedtime: Brush teeth, set the alarm, etc. Do presleep routine the same way every night.
5. Go to bed only when sleepy. Turn out the lights as soon as you get into bed. Assume your preferred alpha sleep position until drowsy, and then assume your preferred omega sleep position.
6. If sleep does not come within a short time (ten minutes, or twenty minutes for seniors), get up and go into a separate room. If none is available, go to another part of the room (separated by a divider, if possible). In the new area occupy yourself with some nonstimulating activity and relaxation exercises until early warning signs of drowsiness occur. At this point quickly return to bed again, assuming your preferred omega sleep position. Return to bed only when you are sleepy.
7. If still not asleep after a brief time, get up again and return to the separate area, remaining there until drowsy again. Repeat this process until you are able to fall asleep and stay asleep. Use

this method if you wake in the night and are unable to fall asleep within ten minutes (twenty minutes for seniors).

8. Avoid daytime naps.

Notes:

The aim of this technique is to break the negative associations that exist between bedroom and sleep, and to turn the bedrooom from a prison to a refuge again.

This procedure takes about ten to twelve weeks to be effective and usually requires professional support to reinforce the ability to carry out the program. There will be an increase of sleepiness and daytime fatigue the first week or so when using this technique. These effects are only temporary and are relieved as sleep capacity at bedtime is regained and difficulty about falling asleep disappears.

Some important errors to avoid in applying this technique are:

1. Failing to get out of bed when unable to fall asleep. (Trying harder to sleep at these times doesn't work and will result in frustration and arousal.)
2. If it is too cold in the new location, it may cause a failure of compliance unless robes and blankets are used.
3. The fear of waking your partner on leaving the bed, or waiting too long to leave. This can be caused by thinking the return of sleep is imminent. If twenty-five minutes or more are spent in getting out of bed at the proper interval, then plan to stay up for twenty-five minutes to make up for this retardation in getting up.
4. Going back to bed too quickly before reaching the desired state of drowsiness. This is caused by a fear that staying up too long will cause too much wakefulness and make you unable to return to sleep.
5. If a nap is absolutely necessary, schedule it before 3 P.M. in the afternoon for forty-five minutes at most.
6. This schedule must be strictly kept on weekends with adherence to the desired waketime. If this is difficult (for the young or for the older socially active persons) oversleeping by one or two hours on Saturday or Sunday is allowed, but this is the limit.

7. In order to facilitate matters on the weekends, plan ahead for activities which will be welcomed and thus make waking easier.
8. Read in bed only if it does not take more than thirty minutes to fall asleep.
9. Use an alarm clock, even a backup alarm, to be able to get up and out easily. Do not oversleep!

References

Lacks, P. *Behavioral Treatment for Persistent Insomnia.* Elmsford, New York: Pergamon Press, 1987.
Bootzin, R. R., and P. M. Nicassio, "Behavioral treatments for insomnia." In Hersen, M., et al., eds. *Progress in Behavior Modification*, vol. 6. New York: Academic Press, 1978, 1–45.
Morin, C. M. *Insomnia: Psychological Assessment and Management.* New York: Guilford Press, 1993.
See also Notes and References for chapter 4.

Sleep Restriction Therapy

1. Maintain a sleep diary for one to two weeks, averaging out the number of hours spent in bed each night.
2. Sleep Restriction Therapy takes an average of ten to twelve weeks to work. Begin the first week by restricting the amount of time spent in bed each night to no more than the average night's sleep you have determined. For example, if you find your average night's sleep totals six hours, be sure that the time you spend in bed each night the first week is only six hours.
3. In no case should the amount of sleep be less than five hours. If less, begin the program by staying in bed for five and a half hours.
4. Each week increase the amount of time spent in bed by fifteen minutes.
5. The aim of this procedure is to reduce the amount of time spent in bed. As a rule, a person who loses sleep spends too much time in bed trying to make up for the loss. This is an error since sleep under these circumstances will be lighter, less refreshing,

and more fragmented. The aim of sleep restriction is to make sleep time in bed limited but, as a result, more efficient.

6. Be sure to schedule sleep time with a specific waketime in the morning. Hold this waketime constant and make lights-out at an appropriate time, in accordance with the total amount of sleep time previously determined. For example, if the best waketime for you is 6 A.M., and your average night's sleep totals six hours, then you begin the program by going to bed no earlier than midnight. If you cannot fall asleep in ten or fifteen minutes, get out of bed and stay up in another room until you are able to fall asleep in ten or fifteen minutes. Most probably with sleep restriction therapy, the bedtime is so delayed that it is relatively easy to fall asleep at a scheduled time.

7. One of the major difficulties of this program is that in the first few weeks there is strong pressure to fall asleep too early. This must be avoided, and for this reason backup professional support is recommended. The program gradually increases the amount of sleep at the rate of fifteen minutes per week. Remember daytime naps, if taken, should be included in the night's sleep total. In no case are they to exceed forty-five minutes, should not be taken unless absolutely necessary, and must occur before 3 P.M. in the afternoon. It is important also to select a reasonable and convenient waketime for yourself and to maintain it throughout the course of the entire program.

References

Spielman, A. J., and P. B. Glovinsky, "A behavioral perspective on insomnia treatment." In Erman, M., ed. *Psychiatric Clinics of North America.* Philadelphia: W. B. Saunders, 1987, 541–553.
Spielman, A. J., P. Saskin, and M. J. Thorpy, "Treatment of chronic insomnia by restriction of time in bed." *Sleep* 1987, 10(1):45–56.

Paradoxical Intention Technique

In Paradoxical Intention Technique, the aim is to prevent obsessional focusing on the necessity of sleep. When sleep is difficult, a person might think the following thought, "I am going to try to stay awake as long as possible and fight off all tendencies to fall asleep." This is paradoxical, since the more one consciously tries to stay awake the more there is a tendency to fall asleep since the arousing concern about sleep is being shunted aside in the effort.

Notes

It is recommended that the paradoxical intention to stay awake be invested with humor, if possible, as "I'm going to set a new world's record for insomnia, and my name will go down in the *Guinness Book of World Records.*"

Reference

Ascher, L. M., and R. M. Turner, "Paradoxical intention and insomnia: an experimental investigation." In *Behavioral Research and Therapy*, vol. 17. 1979, 408–411.

Behavior Therapy in Children

When children have difficulty settling and falling asleep alone in their own beds, some parents are faced with conflicts about how to handle these situations. It is possible to use behavior therapy techniques at such times. Dr. Richard Ferber, the leader in the rapidly burgeoning specialty of pediatric sleep medicine, has devised a desensitization method for dealing with the problem. In brief, Dr. Ferber recommends a scheduled progressive approach where the parent waits a specific amount of time before going into the bedroom to comfort the child. The amount of time the parent waits before entering is progressively lengthened until the child learns to fall asleep alone.

* * *

Ferber's Method of Treating the Child Who Cannot Fall Asleep Alone in the Crib:
   The principle is to desensitize your child to the fear of being alone in its own bed by using a tapered separation schedule.
1. First day: Wait five minutes before going in the child's bedroom if your child is crying and cannot sleep. Comfort your child for two to three minutes and then leave. If more visits are necessary,

wait an additional five minutes for each of the next two visits before going into the room. After the third visit, wait at this level, fifteen minutes, before entering for each later visit until your child falls asleep alone. If child wakes during night, begin again at original level for the night, five minutes, and continue increasing time in five-minute increments as before.

2. Each day thereafter begin first wait with an increase of five minutes above the previous day's first level. Continue with periodic increases—as on first day—until amount of wait time reaches level of the previous day's high level plus the addition of five more minutes. Continue this program with gradual increases of five minutes each day for the initial level and for the maximum level for the night. Do not exceed three increases in any one night. If your child continues wakefulness till about 6:00 A.M., do not continue program but keep child up for the day.

Reference

Ferber, R. *Solve Your Child's Sleep Problems.* New York: Simon and Schuster, 1985.
See also Notes and References for chapter 13.

Cognitive Therapy

Insomniacs have many unrealistic beliefs, attitudes, and expectations about sleeplessness and its treatment.

Cognitive therapy focuses on identifying and altering these faulty thoughts that contribute to continuing maladaptation to sleep difficulties. By correcting these errors of thought, chronic sleep losers are in a better position to overcome their sleep problems. The primary goal is to guide insomniacs to reevaluate the accuracy of their perceptions of their insomnia and its origins and consequences and to replace them with healthier viewpoints.

Some of the tactics are identifying misconceptions about the causes of insomnia (e.g., feeling insomnia is caused by biochemical imbalance); correcting unrealistic sleep expectations (e.g., need to get eight hours of sleep every night); diminish fear of loss of control (e.g., need to control all aspects of life, including sleep); and dispelling myths about good sleep practices (e.g., spending more time in bed will make up for poor or lost sleep).

Reference

Morin, C. M. *Insomnia: Psychological Assessment and Management.* New York: Guilford Press, 1993.

Light Therapy

This is a nondrug treatment of several sleep problems that involve the circadian timing system. The discovery, in the winter type of Seasonal Affective Disorder, that exposure to bright light could reverse the negative effects on SAD victims of diminished daylight in winter, was the springboard for the development of this form of treatment.

The name *phototherapy* was originally given to this treatment, but since this term had already been used to describe a form of treatment for an infant disorder, the term *Light Therapy* (or *Bright Light Therapy*) came into use.

The source of illumination in light therapy is fluorescent lighting. The strength of the lamp is variable. The current level that is generally used is 10,000 lux. Lux is the unit of measurement for illumination and is a measure of the amount of light that the retina of the eye receives. The specific amount of time of exposure, the intensity of the light, and the distance from the light are variables. The person is instructed to look at the lamp briefly every few minutes for a specific length of time at specified times of the day that the treating sleep specialist recommends.

The fluorescent lamps are specially coated to reduce glare and to shut out wavelengths of ultraviolet rays that could damage the corneas of the eyes by causing cataracts. It is strongly advised that bright light therapy be employed only under the supervision of a specialist trained in its use. Some possible side effects are: eyestrain, headaches, dizziness, irritability, and hyperarousal.

Light therapy should not be used where there are retinal or other eye problems that cause sensitivity to light, or where there are drugs being taken or used that also cause sensitivity to light.

The following examples illustrate various degrees of light intensity in our environment.

1. Ordinary room light or twilight indoors   300 to 500 lux
2. Well-lit office   500 to 1000 lux
3. Bright sunny summer day   100,000 lux
4. One-half hour after sunrise on a clear day   10,000 lux

References

Hyman, J. W. *The Light Book*. Los Angeles: Tarcher, 1990.
Rosenthal, N. E. *Seasons of the Mind*. New York: Guilford Press, 1993.
Smyth, A. *SAD: Winter Depression—Who Gets It, What Causes It and How to Cure It*. London: Union, 1990.
Terman, M. "Light Therapy." In Kryger, M. H., Roth, T., and Dement, W. C., eds. *Principles and Practice of Sleep Medicine*. Philadelphia: W. B. Saunders, 1989, 717–722.
See also Notes and References for chapter 6.

Notes and References

The reader who is seeking more knowledge about sleep and insomnia is currently in an especially propitious position. For those who wish to avail themselves of resources beyond the popular books on these topics, there now exist a number of general volumes published by sleep specialists which contain much information presented in a way that is not too technical nor abstruse. These books, primarily for students of sleep medicine or scientists in related fields who are interested in sleep and its disorders, cover the topic of sleep comprehensively and are written in a manner that can, in the main, be understood by the intelligent layperson.

The following list of recommended books is presented in a graded scale with the most general and least technical volumes cited first, followed by those of increasing levels of expertise and complexity:

Hobson, A. J. *Sleep.* (New York: Scientific American Library, 1989.)

Aronoff, M. S. *Sleep and Its Secrets.* (New York: Plenum Press, 1991.)

Lamberg, L. *AMA Guide to Better Sleep.* (New York: Random House, 1984.) Popular. Old but inclusive.

Hauri, P. and S. Linde. *No More Sleepless Nights.* (New York: Wiley, 1990.)

Moorcroft, W. H. *Sleep, Dreaming and Sleep Disorders.* (Lanham, MD: University Press of America, 1989.)

Webb, W. *Sleep, the Gentle Tyrant* 2nd ed. (Boston: Anker, 1992.) Popular review of advances in the field.

Riley, T. L. *Clinical Aspects of Sleep and Sleep Disturbance.* (Boston: Butterworth, 1985.)

Parkes, J. D. *Sleep and Its Disorders.* (Philadelphia: W. B. Saunders, 1985.)

Anch, A. M., et al., eds. *Sleep: A Scientific Perspective.* (Englewood Cliffs, N.J.: Prentice-Hall, 1988.)

Mendelson, W. B. *Human Sleep.* (New York: Plenum Press, 1987.)

A professional volume devoted entirely to the topic of insomnia is: Kales, A., and J. Kales. *Evaluation and Treatment of Insomnia.* (New York: Oxford University Press, 1984.)

The recent publication of Kryger, M. H., T. Roth, and W. C. Dement, eds. *Principles and Practice of Sleep Medicine.* (Philadelphia: W. B. Saunders, 1989), a comprehensive textbook available in one volume, gives definitive, up-to-date coverage of the field of sleep medicine. Although designed for professionals in the field, it can be of use for those seeking authoritative data on the specialized range of topics germane to sleep. For those whose interest, informational hunger, and curiosity are not daunted by its technological detail, it can provide nuggets of knowledge and knowing answers about sleep and sleep disorders.

In addition to this textbook the following volumes are also of use as references: Williams, R. L., I. Karacan, and C. Moore, eds. *Sleep Disorders: Diagnosis and Treatment,* 2nd ed. (New York: Wiley, 1988), an authoritative review of the major topics of sleep and sleep medicine, with a succinct survey of pertinent research articles. Reite, M. L., K. E. Nagel, J. R. Ruddy. *Concise Guide to Evaluation and Management of Sleep Disorders.* (Washington, D.C.: American Psychiatric Press, 1990), is a compact presentation of topics on sleep and sleep disorders, presented in an almost outline form. Chokroverty, S., ed. *Sleep Disorders Medicine.* (Boston: Butterworth-Heinemann, 1994); and Thorpy, M. J., ed. *Handbook of Sleep Disorders.* (New York: Marcel Dekker, 1990.) Both these latter two volumes contain comprehensive articles on topics of sleep medicine.

Thorpy, M., and J. Yager, *The Encyclopedia of Sleep and Sleep Disorders.* (New York: Facts on File, 1990); and Carskadon, M. *Encyclopedia of Sleep and Dreaming.* (New York: Macmillan, 1993), are pithy A–Z encyclopedias.

* * *

Rounding out the general review picture are a number of articles published in journals, or as parts of larger volumes, that provide current summations of sleep and sleep disorders. Since most of these articles were written for predominantly professional readers who were not specifically specialists in sleep medicine, they are fairly accessible for the lay reader. Presented in alphabetical order, they are:

Gillin, J. C., and W. F. Byerly, "The diagnosis and management of insomnia." *NEJM* 1990; 322(4): 239–248.

Madow, L., ed. "Sleep disorders." (Special issue) *Psychiatric Annals* 1987; 17:430–490.

Manfredi, R. L., A. Vgontzas, and A. Kales. "An update on sleep disorders." *Bull. Menninger Clinic* 1989; 53:250–273.

Reite, M., "Sleep and sleep disorders." In Simons, R.C., ed. *Understanding Human Behavior in Health and Illness, 3rd ed.* (Baltimore: Williams and Wilkins, 1985); 569–585.

"Sleep Disorders." In Hales, A. J., and A. J. Frances, eds. *APA Annual Review, vol. 4.* 1985; Washington, D.C.: American Psychiatric Press; 259–394.

Sleep Disorders. In Psychiatric Practice. Psychiatric Medicine 1986; 4(2): Longwood, Florida: Ryandic.

* * *

The following abbreviations will be used in individual chapter notes. For Kryger, Roth, and Dement, *Principles and Practice of Sleep Medicine: "Principles And Practice."*

For Williams, Karacan, and Moore, *Sleep Disorders,* 2nd ed. "Williams 2nd ed."

Chapter 1

Hartmann, E., et al. "Psychological differences between long and short sleepers." *Arch. Gen. Psychiat.* 1972; 26:463–468.

A discussion of the insomniac without objective findings can be found in Mendelson, W. B., et al. "A psychophysiological study of insomnia." *Psychiatr. Res.* 1986; 19:267–284.

The epidemiological patterns of insomnia are covered in a series of basic papers: Bixler, E. O., A. Kales, et al. "Prevalence of sleep disorders in the Los Angeles metropolitan area." *Am. J. Psychiatr.* 1979; 136: 1257–1262. Lugaresi, E., et al., "Good and poor sleepers: an epidemiological survey of the San Marino population." In Guilleminault, C., and E. Lugaresi, eds. *Sleep Wake Disorders.* (New York: Raven Press, 1983) 1–12. Karacan, I., J. I. Thornby, M. Anch, et al. "Prevalence of sleep disturbance in a primarily urban Florida county." *Soc. Sci. Med.* 1976; 10:239–244. Thornby, J. I., I. Karacan, et al. "Subjective reports of sleep disturbance in a Houston metropolitan health survey." *Sleep Res.* 1977; 6:180. See also Kales, A., and J. Kales. *op. cit.,* ch. 4.

For the story of a total nonsleeper, see feature article *San Francisco Chronicle,* Apr. 22, 1986.

The relationship of insomnia to mood and performance is dealt with in: Bonnet, M. H., "Effect of sleep disruption on sleep, performance, and mood." *Sleep* 1985; 8:11–19, Dinges, D. F., and R. J. Broughton, eds.

Sleep and Alertness: Chronobiological, Behavioral, and Medical Aspects of Napping. (New York: Raven Press, 1989); Stepanski, E., et al. "Daytime alertness in patients with chronic insomnia. . . ." *Sleep* 1988; 11(1):54–60.

Stress in relationship to insomnia is discussed in Healy, E. S., A. Kales, L. J. Monroe, et al. "Onset of insomnia: role of life-stress events." *Psychosom. Med.* 1981; 43:439–451.

Excellent coverage of the various medical causes of insomnia is to be found in *Principles and Practice,* ch. 50, and Williams 2nd ed., chs. 13, 14. "ABC of sleep disorders." *BMJ* 1993; 306(6891):1532–1535 is a summary of this topic.

Concerning sleep and personality: Stepanski, E., et al. "Sleep and personality characteristics of patients and subjects with chronic complaints of insomnia." *Sleep Res.* 1987; 16:439, Hauri, P. "A cluster analysis of insomnia." *Sleep* 1983; 6(4):326–338, de la Pena, A. "Toward a psychophysiological conceptualization of insomnia." In *Williams* 2nd ed., 101–143. See also A. Kales, and J. Kales, *op. cit.* chs. 4, 5: 41–133.

Concerning milk allergy as a cause of insomnia in children, see Kahn, A., et al. "Intolerance to cow's milk can be a hidden cause of chronic insomnia in children." *Sleep Res.* 1990; 19:327.

Roth. T., et al. "The effects of noise during sleep on the sleep patterns of different age groups." *Can. Psychiat. Assoc. J.* 1972; 17:196–201.

Chapter 2

See *Principles and Practice,* chs. 4–6 for a discussion of the topics of the evolution of sleep and animal sleep.

Borbely, A., *Secrets of Sleep.* (New York: Basic Books, 1986), ch. 7, has a good brief discussion of animal sleep; as does Moorcroft, W. H., *op. cit.* ch. 3.

See *Principles and Practice,* chs. 11–13, for an extended coverage of chronobiology. A basic book on the topic is Moore-Ede, M. C., F. M. Sulzman, and C. A. Fuller, *The Clocks That Time Us: Physiology of the Circadian Timing System.* (Cambridge: Harvard University Press, 1982.)

"ABC of sleep disorders." *BMJ* 1993; 306(6874):383–385. Functions of sleep: conservation of energy; restoration. Succinct coverage of theories.

Hans Berger was the father of the EEG study of the electrical activity of the brain and its graphic patterns.

Loomis, A. L., E. N. Harvey, and G. A. Hobart. "Cerebral states during sleep as studied by human brain potentials." *J. Exp. Psychol.* 1937; 21:127–144, first described EEG patterns in sleep.

Aserinsky, E., and N. Kleitman. "Regularly occurring periods of eye motility, and concomitant phenomena, during sleep." *Science* 1953; 118:273–274, is the original paper on the discovery of REM sleep. The correlations between eye movements, sleep, and dreaming was shown originally in: Dement, W. C., and N. Kleitman. "Cyclic variations in EEG during sleep and their relation to eye movements, body motility and dreaming." *Electroenceph. Neurophysiol.* 1957; 9:673–690.

The depth of sleep stages is the theme of the basic paper, Rechtschaffen, A., Hauri, P., and M. Zeitlin. "Auditory awakening thresholds in REM and NREM sleep stages." *Percep. Mot. Skills.* 1966; 22:927–942.

Chapter 4

Freedman, R. R. and H. L. Satler. "Physiological and psychological factors in sleep-onset insomnia." *J. Abnorm. Psychol.* 1982; 91:380–389.

See "Sleep and Anxiety," in Williams 2nd ed., 189–214. For the relationship between panic disorders and sleep, Uhde, T. W., P. P. Roy-Byrne, J. C. Gillin, et al. "The sleep of patients with panic disorder." *Psychiatr. Res.* 1984; 12:251–259. See also the following: *J. Clin. Psychiat.* July 1991; 52 Suppl. contains articles on relation of insomnia to anxiety varieties; Mellman, T. A., and T. W. Uhde. "Sleep panic attacks." *Amer. J. Psychiatr.* 1989; 146:1204–1207; Glaubman, H., et al. "Sleep of chronic posttraumatic patients." *J. Traum. Stress. Stud.* 1990; 3:255–263; Hauri, P. J., et al. "Sleep in patients with spontaneous panic attacks." *Sleep* 1989; 12:323–337.

A special case of sleep onset insomnia occurs in young depressives. This is in contrast to the usual situation of depression, where the pattern is usually that of an early A.M. insomnia. For insomnia patterns in depression in the younger age groups, see Lahmeyer, H. W., et al. "Sleep in depressed adolescents." *Am. J. Psychiatr.* 1983; 140:1150–1153. It is important to check for signs of depression (recent losses, mood changes, and vegetative symptoms such as lowered libido, weight loss, and insomnia) in young depressives who only seem to manifest the complaint of initial insomnia.

For discussion of this important topic, see the following: Hauri, P., and J. Fisher. "Persistent psychophysiologic (learned) insomnia." *Sleep* 1986; 9(1):38–53. Kales, A., and J. Kales, *op. cit.*, 118–133, and Williams 2nd ed., 36–42.

For a description of the technique of stimulus control, Bootzin, R. R., and P. Nicassio. "Behavioral treatment in insomnia." In Hersen, R., et al., eds. *Progress in Behavior Modification, vol. 6.* (New York: Academic Press, 1978). See also, Hauri, P., ed. *Case Studies in Insomnia.* (New York: Plenum Press, 1990); Part I, 19–86. For other behavioral techniques dealing with this condition, see Kales, A., and J. Kales, *op. cit.*, 231–240.

Chapter 5

Hauri, P., and D. R. Hawkins. "Alpha-delta sleep." *EEG Clin. Neurophysiol.* 1973; 34:233–237. Saskin, P., H. Moldofsky, and F. A. Lue. "Sleep and post-traumatic rheumatic pain modulation disorder (fibrositis syndrome)." *Psychosom. Med.* 1986; 48:319–323.

For discussion of larynx spasm in sleep, see Thorpy, M. J., and F. Aloe. "Choking during sleep." *Sleep Res.* 1989; 18:313–314.

For other sources of middle insomnia: Krupp, L. B. "Sleep disturbance in Chronic Fatigue Syndrome." *J. Psychosom. Res.* 1993; 37(4):325–331, a medical condition with sleep effects currently under intense investigation.

Pearce, J. M. S., "Exploding head syndrome." *Lancet* 1988; 11:270–271, presentation of a middle insomnia cause, occurring mainly in older women.

Chapter 6

For excellent discussions of the relationship of insomnia, and sleep and depression see the following sources: Kales, A., and J. Kales, *op. cit.* ch. 11, 282–307. Hales, R. E., and Frances, A., eds. *Amer. Psychiatr. Assoc., Ann. Rev., vol. 4.* (Washington, D.C.: American Psychiatric Press, 1985); 341–351. Gillin, J. C., N. Sitaram, T. Wehr, et al. "Sleep and affective illness." In Post, R. M., and Ballenger, J. C., eds. *Neurobiology of Mood Disorders.* (Baltimore: William and Wilkins, 1984); 157–189. Gillin, C., et al., "Successful prediction of depressed normal and insomniac patients by EEG sleep data." *Arch. Gen. Psychiat.* 1979; 36:85–90; also Reynolds, C. F., and Kupfer, D. J., "Sleep research and affective illness: State of the art circa 1987." *Sleep* 1987; 10:199–215.

In addition to utilization of placebo schedule and group support for drug withdrawal, stimulus control technique can be of use. See discussion of this technique in ch. 8, and Appendix this volume.

Thorough coverage of seasonal affective disorder is found in the following volumes: Rosenthal, N. E. *Seasons of the Mind.* (New York: Guilford Press, 1989.) Rosenthal, N. E. and M. Blehar, eds. *Seasonal Affective Disorder and Phototherapy.* (New York: Guilford Press, 1989.) Silverstone, T., and C. Thompson, eds. *Seasonal Affective Disorder.* (London: CNS Clinical Neuroscience, 1989.)

Since carbohydrate craving is a cardinal symptom of SAD, it is no surprise that it also makes its appearance in the late afternoon, as expected by the biphasic pattern of sleep.

Wehr, T., et al. "Contrast between symptoms of summer depression and winter depression." *J. Affect. Disord.* 1991; 23(4):173–183.

Chapter 8

Karacan, I., et al. "Dose-related sleep disturbances induced by coffee and caffeine." *Clin. Pharm. Therapeut.* 1976; 20:682–689; and Bonnet, M. H., and D. L. Arrand. "Caffeine use as a model of acute and chronic insomnia." *Sleep* 1992; 15(6):526–536.

Soldatos, C. R., et al. "Cigarette smoking associated with sleep difficulty." *Science* 1980; 207:551–552.

Chapter 9

For discussion of the important topic of snoring, see *Principles and Practice*, ch. 53.

Aspects of yawning are covered in the three citations: Bell, L. A., "Boredom and the Yawn." *Rev. of Existent Psychol. and Psychiatr.* 1980; 17:91–100. Lehman, H. E., "Yawning: a homeostatic reflex and its psychological significance." *Bulletin of the Menninger Clinic* 1979; 43:123–136. Garma, L., and H. J. Aubin. "Yawning: a vigilance-enhancing factor?" *Sleep. Res.* 1989; 18:4.

Jacobson, E., *You Can Sleep Well.* (London: Whittlesey House, 1938); and *Progressive Relaxation.* (Chicago: University of Chicago Press, 1929.)

Chapter 10

For an extensive review of the history of the development of sleeping pills, see Hartmann, E., *The Sleeping Pill.* (New Haven: Yale University Press, 1978.)

For discussions of hypnotics, see Hartmann, E., reference above, as well as Mendelson, W. B. *The Use and Misuse of Sleeping Pills.* (New York: Plenum Press, 1980.) "Consensus conference: drugs and insomnia: The use of medications to promote sleep." *JAMA* 1984; 251:2410–2414. Roth, T., T. Roehrs, and F. Zorick. "Pharmacological treatment of sleep disorders." In Williams 2nd ed., 373–395. Nicholson, A. N., C. M. Bradley, and P. A. Pascoe. In *Principles and Practice*, 228–236. Mellinger, G. D., M. B. Balter, and E. H. Uhlenhuth. "Insomnia and Its Treatment." *Arch. Gen. Psychiatr.* 1985; 42:225–232; and *J. Clin. Psychiatr.* June 1992; 53 Suppl; 3–45; *J. Clin. Psychiatr.* Dec. 1992; 53 Suppl; 3–87; these two articles are good up-to-date reviews. Also Mendelson, W. B. in Thorpy, *op. cit.*, 737–753.

Chloral hydrate has recently been alleged to be implicated in tumor formation in children. Until this is evaluated, caution should be exercised in its use.

Benzodiazepine Dependence, Toxicity, and Abuse. (Washington, D.C.: American Psychiatric Press, 1990), is a good, brief discussion of uses and actions of the BDZs.

For rebound effects in short acting BDZs, Kales, A., et al., "Rebound insomnia and rebound anxiety: a review." *Pharmacology* 1983; 26:121–137.

Chapter 11

"ABC of sleep disorders." *BMJ* 1993; 306:448–451. Good summary of topic of circadian rhythms. For more professional review of topic, see Wagner, D. R., in Thorpy, *op. cit.*, 531–550.

For jet lag, see Coleman, R. M. *Wide Awake at 3:00 AM: By Choice or By Chance.* (New York: Freeman. *Principles and Practice,* 1986) ch. 32.

Weitzman, E. D., C. A. Czeisler, R. M. Coleman, et al. "Delayed sleep phase syndrome." *Arch. Gen. Psychiatr.* 1981; 38:737–746. Czeisler, C. A., et al. "Chrono-therapy: Resetting the circadian clocks of patients with delayed sleep-phase insomnia." *Sleep* 1981; 4:1–21. These papers deal with delayed sleep phase syndrome and the chronotherapy technique.

For shift work, see Johnson, L. C., et al, eds. *Biological Rhythms, Sleep and Shift Work.* (New York: SP Medicine and Scientific Books, 1981). *Principles and Practice,* ch. 33. Czeisler, C. A., et al. "Exposure to bright light and darkness to treat physiological maladaption to night work." *NEJM* 1990; 322:1253–9.

Chapter 12

For descriptions of the apneas, see *Principles and Practice,* chs. 53–61, and Williams 2nd ed., ch. 4; and Guilleminault, C., and W. C. Dement, eds. *Sleep Apnea Syndromes.* (New York: Alan R. Liss, 1978); and Bradley, T. D., and E. A. Phillipson, "Central sleep apnea." *Clin. Ches. Med.* 1992; 13(3):493–505.

For surgical techniques in treating apnea, see the excellent discussions, which include graphic illustrations, in Fairbanks, D.N.F., et al., *Snoring and Obstructive Sleep Apnea.* (New York: Raven Press, 1987).

The myth of Ondine's curse is described in Colp, C., R. Schneider, and D. Altarac, "Ondine's curse revisited." *New York State J. Med.* 1989; 89:228–230. Tamerin, F., R. J. Goldberg, and R. D. Brandstetter, "The tale of Ondine: A curse, a kiss, a clasp, and a comment." *New York State J Med.* 1989; 89:146–198. Girandoux, J., *Ondine, A Romantic Fantasy in Three Acts.* (New York: Samuel French, 1956.)

For an excellent volume on narcolepsy, see Roth, B. *Narcolepsy and Hypersomnia.* Basel: 1980; also *Principles and Practice*, ch. 34, and Williams 2nd ed., ch. 6.

For restless legs and PLMS, see Montplaisir, J., and R. Godbout. "Restless legs and periodic movements during sleep," in *Principles and Practice*, ch. 43. Williams 2nd ed., ch. 5. Walters, A. S. "Clinical presentation and neuropharmacology of restless leg syndrome." In *Clin. Neuropharmacol.* 1987; 10:225–237. Coleman, R. M., C. P. Pollak, and E. D. Weitzman. "Periodic movements in sleep (nocturnal myoclonus): relation to sleep disorders." *Am. Neurol.* 1980; 8:416–421. Guilleminault, C., ed. *Sleeping and Waking Disorders.* (Menlo Park, Cal.: Addison-Wesley, 1982.)

Chapter 13

The two major books on children's sleep are: Ferber, R. *Solve Your Child's Sleep Problems.* (New York: Simon and Schuster, 1985); and Guilleminault, C., ed. *Sleep and Its Disorders in Children.* New York: Raven Press, 1987.) The first is a popular book, but so fundamental, extensive, and authoritative that it has already become a classic. The second volume is a collection of excellent articles on the topic. See also: Ferber, R., in Thorpy, *op. cit.*, 435–455; and also Gillin, J. C., ed. "The ontogeny of sleep disorders in childhood;" et al., *Amer. Psychiatr. Assoc. Annual Review vol. 4, Psychiatric Update* (Washington, D.C.: American Psychiatric Press, 1985) 329–340.

The parasomnias are described and discussed in: Mahowald, M. W., and Ettinger, M. G. "Things that go bump in the night: The parasomnias revisited." *J. Clin. Neurophysiol.* 1990; 7:119–143. Hartmann, E., et al. "Bruxism: Personality traits and other characteristics." *Sleep Res.* 1987; 16:350. Kales, A., et al. "Sleep disorders: insomnia, sleepwalking, night terrors, nightmares, and enuresis." *Ann. Int. Med.* 1987; 106(4):582–592.

Childhood-onset insomnia is the topic of two papers: Hauri, P., and E. Olmstead, "Childhood-onset insomnia." *Sleep* 1980; 3:59–65. Regestein, Q. R., and P. Reich, "Incapacitating childhood-onset insomnia." *Compr. Psychiatr.* 1983; 24:244–248.

Chapter 14

The following two references deal, in an overall way, with sleep and sleep disturbances in the older population. These two excellent volumes, neither of which is too technical, are: Hartmann, E. *The Sleep Book.*

(Glenview, Ill.: Scott, Foresman 1987.) Morgan, K. *Sleep and Aging.* (Baltimore: Johns Hopkins Press, 1987.)

See also Albarede, J. L., et al. *Sleep Disorders and Insomnia in the Elderly.* (New York: Springer, 1993.) Collected special articles on senior sleep problems; technical.

The following references are general comprehensive articles on the topic: Vitielo, M. V., and P. N. Prinz, "Aging and sleep disorders." In Williams 2nd ed., 293–312. Bliwise, D. L., "Normal Aging." In *Principles and Practice*, 24–29. Billiard, M., and A. Besset, "Insomnia in the elderly." In Emser, W., D. Kurtz, and W. B. Webb, eds. *Sleep, Aging and Related Disorders/Symposium 3 on Sleep Disorders.* (New York: Karger 1987), 98–110. Dement, W., Richardson, G., et al. "Changes of sleep with age." In Finch, C., Schneider, E. L., eds. *Handbook of the Biology of Aging*, 2nd ed. (New York: Van Nostrand Reinhold 1985) 692–717. Regestein, Q., "Sleep and insomnia in the elderly." *J. Geriatr. Psychiatr.* 1980; 13:153–171.

The following references are excellent summary articles. Prinz, P. N., M. V. Vitiello, M. A. Raskind, and M. J. Thorpy. "Geriatrics: sleep disorders and aging." *NEJM* 1990; 323(8):520–526. Miles, L. E., and W. Dement, "Sleep and Aging." *Sleep* 1980; 3(2):119–220. Reynolds, C. F., Kupfer, D. J., et al. "The sleep of healthy seniors: A revisit." *Sleep* 1985; 8:20–29.

See Kahn, E., C. Fisher, and L. Lieberman. "Sleep characteristics of the human aged female." *Compr. Psychiatr.* 1970; 11:274–278; and Bliwise, D. L. "Factors related to sleep quality in healthy elderly women." *Psychol. Aging* 1992; 7(1):83–88.

For characteristics of depression in the older age group, see Blazer, D., "The diagnosis of depression in the elderly." *J. Amer. Ger. Soc.* 1980; 28:52–58. Rapp, S. R., and Vrana, S. "Substituting nonsomatic for somatic symptoms in the diagnosis of depression in elderly male medical patients." *J. Amer. Psychiat.* 1989; 146(9):1197–1200. Young, R. C. "Pharmacological treatment of depression in the elderly." *Psychiatr. Ann.* 1990; 20:102–107.

Bliwise, D. L., "Sleep in normal aging and dementia." *Sleep* 1993; 16(1):40–81.

For hypnotic use in the elderly, see ch. 11, this volume. For an excellent discussion of hypnotic use in various sleep conditions, especially the elderly, see Moran, M. S., T. L. Thompson, and A. S. Nies. "Sleep disorders in the elderly." *Am. J. Psychiatr.* 1988; 145; 11:1369–1378.

Chapter 15

Reference Dunkell, S. *Sleep Positions.* (New York: Morrow, 1977.)
For the early works on sleep positions, see the following references.

Adler, A., *The Individual Psychology of Alfred Adler*. (New York: Basic Books, 1956), 221–222. Schalit, S. "Ueber Schlafstellungen." *Internatl. Ztschrift. f. Indiv. Psychol.* 1925; 3:97–103. Thorner, H. "Die Koerperstellung im Schlaf." *Nervenarzt* 1931; 4:197–206. Johnson, H. M., et al. "In what position do healthy people sleep?" *JAMA* 1930; 94:2058–2062. Stradling, R., and D. A. Laird. "Further data on the handedness of sleep." *J. Abnorm. Soc. Psychol.* 1934; 29:462–464.

Schuetz, F. reported on sleep positions in the *Lancet* Dec. 10, 1941; 241:774–775 and made the observation, ". . . that this [sleep position] was definitely characteristic for each individual. The individual seldom varied the position and when he did he was fully conscious that he had made a change. . . ." Leak, W. N., commenting on this in the *Lancet*, Jan. 3, 1942; 1:26, affirmed this persistence and singularity when ". . . an accident prevented me from lying on my right side. I noticed how difficult it was to accommodate myself to lying on my left side and wondered why. . . ."

Beyond their observations and insights, it interested me that although these accounts were written a few weeks after Pearl Harbor, they contain no remarks about war stress and its effects on the patients these physicians were seeing. It is also remarkable that there is no mention of the highly stressful and abnormal mass underground settings in which Londoners and the inhabitants of other cities had to sleep during war and siege. Dunkell, S. *LoveLives*. (New York: Morrow, 1978.) p. 135.

Domino, G., and S. A. Bohn, "Hypnagogic exploration: Sleep positions and personality." *J. Clin. Psychol.* 1980; 36(3):760–762.

In 1983, Joseph De Koninck and his Ottawa group began their studies on sleep positions utilizing time lapse photography. See articles: De Koninck, J., P. Gagnon, and S. Lallier, "Sleep positions in the young adult and the subjective quality of sleep." *Sleep* 1983; 6:52–59. De Koninck, J., D. Lorrain, and P. Gagnon. "An expanded picture of the ontogenesis of sleep positions in the human." In Koella, W. P., ed. *Sleep '86*. 1988; New York: Gustav Fischer. Lorrain, D., et al. "Sleep positions and postural shifts in elderly persons." *Percept. Mot. Skills* 1986; 63(2):352–354. Lorrain, D., et al. "Sleep positions in psychophysiological insomnia." *Sleep Res.* 1988; 17:215. DeKoninck, J., D. Lorrain, and P. Gagnon. "Sleep positions and position shifts in five age groups: An ontogenetic picture." *Sleep* 1992; 15(2):143–149.

Dzvonik, M. L., et al. "Body position changes and periodic movements in sleep." *Sleep* 1986; 9:484–491, shows correlations between movements during sleep and position.

In the last decade dozens of articles have appeared on correlations between sleep position and sleep apnea. Among the many references are the following: Lloyd, S. R. "The sleep position effect in sleep apnea as a continuous variable." *Sleep Res.* 1988; 17:214. Miles, L., and A. Bailey, "Evaluation of sleep apnea treatment must be related to sleeping position." *Sleep Res.* 1990; 19:256. Orr, W. C., et al. "Modulation of central sleep apnea by sleeping position." *Sleep Res.* 1986; 15:152. Kavey, N. B., et al. "Sleeping position and sleep apnea syndrome." *Amer. J. Otolaryngol.* 1985; 6:373–377. Pevernagie, D. A., and J. W. Shepard, "Relations between sleep stage, posture and effective nasal CPAP levels in OSA." *Sleep* 1992; 15(2):162–167. Solow, B., et al. "Head posture in obstructive sleep apnea." *Eur. J. Orthod.* 1993; 15(2):107–114.

In 1984, Rosalind Cartwright began publication of a series of papers on correlations between sleep apnea and changes in sleep position, as well as efforts to correct the problem. See for example, Cartwright, R. D. "Effect of sleep position on sleep apnea severity." *Sleep* 1984; 7:110–114. Cartwright, R. D., et al., "Sleep position training as treatment for sleep apnea." *Sleep* 1985; 8:87–94. Cartwright, R. D., et al. "Comparing two treatments for positional sleep apnea: TRD and posture alarm." *Sleep Res.* 1990; 19:202; and two other papers by Cartwright, viz. "A comparative study of treatments for positional sleep apnea." *Sleep* 1991; 14(6):546–552; "The effects of sleep posture and sleep stage on apnea frequency." *Sleep* 1991; 14(4):351–353.

A flood of articles on the relation of prone sleep position and Sudden Infant Death Syndrome has appeared in the last years. Some of these are: Poets, C. F., and D. P. Southall. "Prone sleeping and sudden infant death syndrome" [editorial]. *NEJM* 1993; 329(6):425–426. Ponsonby, A. L., et al. "Factors potentiating the risk of sudden infant death syndrome associated with the prone position." *NEJM* 1993; 329(6):377–382.

Hume, I. N., *Martin's Hundred.* (New York: Knopf, 1982) 284–291. Tells the "Granny" story.

Wiley, B. I., *Common Soldier in the Civil War.* (New York: Grosset and Dunlap, 1951.)

Chapter 16

Rhoads, N. P., et al. "Marital status of patients with sleep disorders." *Sleep Res.* 1989; 18:295.

For correlations between insomnia and sexuality, see Wise, T. N. "Difficulty falling asleep after coitus." *Med. Aspects of Hum. Sexuality* 1981; 15(3):144–158.

In my clinical practice I have noted some provocative connections between sleep and sex. For example it has been cited to me that the experience of orgasm is associated with an "out of the world" momentary loss of consciousness during climax. I speculate that what occurs is a "micro-sleep" at the time of ultimate orgastic pleasure.

The role of sexual fantasy during the preorgastic phase is another example of a clinical phenomenon that may reveal the close links between sex and sleep. As orgasm is approached conscious sexual fantasies, when present, become dreamlike and then disappear. Do these fantasies have ties to the process of dreaming, do they facilitate orgasm, and do they in fact become dream phenomena?

I am studying these phenomena and their further implications, to see whether they are in actuality forms of sleep and dreaming.

Chapter 17

For references on correlations between sleep and pregnancy, see Moorcroft, W. H., op. cit., 119–121.

Karacan, et al. "Characteristics of sleep patterns during late pregnancy and the postpartum period." Amer. J. Obst. Gyn. 1968; 101:579–586.

For correlations between menstrual cycle and sleep, see Mauri, M., R. L. Reid, and A. W. MacLean. "Sleep in the premenstrual phase." Acta Psychiatr. Scand. 1988; 78:82–86. Wagner, D. R., M. L. Moline, and C. P. Pollak. "Internal desynchronization of circadian rhythms in free-running young females occurs at specific phases of the menstrual cycle." Sleep Res. 1989; 18:449. Schultz, K. J., and D. Koulack. "Dream effect and the menstrual cycle." J. Nerv. Ment. Dis. 1980; 168:436–438. Severino, S. K., W. Bucci, and M. L. Creelman. "Cyclical changes in emotional information processing in sleep and dreams." J. Am. Acad. Psychoanal. 1989; 17(4):555–578.

Principles and Practice, ch. 75 has excellent coverage of the topic of penile erections and sleep. See also, Hirshkowitz, M., I. Karacan, and J. W. Howell. "Sleep-related erections, erectile dysfunction, and marital status." Sleep Res. 1989; 18:337.

See also, Ware, J. C., "Evaluation of impotence-monitoring periodic penile erections during sleep." Psychiatr. Clin. No. Amer. 1987; 10:675–686; and Thase, M. E., et al. "Diminished nocturnal penile tumescence in depression . . ." Biol. Psychiatr. 1992; 31(11):1136–1142.

Chapter 18

For general background information on dreams and dream thinking, see the following: Wolman, B. B., ed. Handbook of Dreams. (New York: Van Nostrand Reinhold, 1979.) Arkin, A. M., J. S. Antrobus, and S. Ellman, eds. The Mind in Sleep, 2nd ed. (Hillsdale, N.J.: Lawrence Erlbaum Associates, 1986.) Foulkes, D. A Grammar of Dreams. (New York: Basic

Books, 1978.) Bootzin, R. R., et al., eds. *Sleep and Cognition*. (Hyattsville, Md.: American Psychological Press, 1990.)

Additionally, see Wollman, M. C., and J. S. Antrobus, "Sleeping and waking thought: Effects of external stimulation." *Sleep* 1986; 9(3): 438–448. Williams 2nd ed., ch. 12. Moorcroft, W. H., *op. cit.*, ch 5. Witkin, H., and H. B. Lewis, *Experimental Studies of Dreaming*. (New York: Random House, 1967), is a classic early work. Antrobus, J. S., and M. Bertini, *The Neuropsychology of Sleep and Dreaming*. (Hillsdale, N.J.: Lawrence Erlbaum Associates, 1992), has chapters on bizarreness, lucid dreams, neurophysiology, et al.

Dreaming (New York: Human Science Press), a new journal devoted to dreaming, is published quarterly by the Association for the Study of Dreams. It began with the March 1991 issue. Articles on topics like dream contents, meanings, and dreams and personality are featured.

Rechtschaffen, A. "The single mindedness and isolation of dreams." *Sleep* 1978; 1:97–109.

Nielson, T. A., et al. "Pain in dreams." *Sleep* 1993; 16(5):490–498.

Cipolli, C., et al. "Bizarreness effect in dream recall." *Sleep* 1993; 16(2):163–170.

For the classic paper on effects of divorce and depression on dreams, see Cartwright, R., et al. "Broken dreams: a study of the effects of divorce and depression on dream content." *Psychiatrist* 1984; 47:251–259. Also, see Cartwright, R. D. "REM sleep characteristics during and after mood-disturbing events." *Arch. Gen. Psychiatr.* 1983; 40:197–201.

Brink, S. G., and J. A. Allen. "Dreams of anorexic and bulimic women . . ." J. Anal. Psychol. 1992; 37(3):275–297.

Posttraumatic stress disorder and dreams are covered in the following references: Burstein, A. "Posttraumatic flashbacks, dream disturbances, and mental imagery." *J. Clin. Psychiatr.* 1985; 46:374–378. Ross, R. J., et al. "Sleep disturbance as the hallmark of posttraumatic stress disorder." *Am. J. Psychiatr.* 1980; 146(6):697–707. Wolf, M. E., and A. D. Mosnaim, *Posttraumatic Stress Disorder: Etiology, Phenomenology, and Treatment.* (Washington D.C.: American Psychiatric Press, 1990.) Hefez, A., L. Metz, and P. Lavie, "Long term effects of extreme situational stress on sleep and dreaming." *Am. J. Psychiatr.* 1987; 144:344–347.

Hall, C., and R. Van de Castle. *The Content Analysis of Dreams*. (Norwalk, Conn.: Appleton-Century-Crofts, 1986), ch. 16. Hall, C. S., W. Domhoff, et al. "The dreams of college men and women in 1950 and 1980: A comparison of dream contents and sex differences." *Sleep* 1982; 5(2): 188–194.

For description of "The Hag," see Hufford, D. *The Terror That Comes in the Night*. (Philadelphia: University of Pennsylvania Press, 1982.)

Hobson, J. A., and R. W. McCarley, "The brain as a dream state generator: An activation-synthesis hypothesis of the dream process." *Am. J. Psychiatr.* 1977; 134:1335–1348. Hobson, J. A. *The Dreaming Brain* (New York: Basic Books, 1988.)

Concerning REM behavior disorder, see Schenck, C. H., S. R. Bundlie, A. L. Patterson, and M. W. Mahowald, "REM sleep behavior disorder." *JAMA* 1987; 257:1786–1789. Mahowald, M. W., and C. H. Schenck, *Principles and Practice.* 389–401.

Other contemporary dream theories are to be found in the following works. Foulkes, D. *Dreaming: A Cognitive-Psychological Analysis.* (Hillsdale, N.J.: Lawrence Erlbaum Associates, 1985.) Foulkes, D. "A cognitive-psychological model of dream production." *Sleep* 1982; 5(2):169–186. F. Crick, and G. Mitchison, "The function of dream sleep." *Nature* 1983; 304:111–114. Koukkou, M., and D. Lehman. "REM sleep dreams and the activation-synthesis hypothesis." *Br. J. Psychiatr.* 1983; 142:221–231.

"ABC of sleep disorders." *BMJ* 1993; 306(6883):993–995. Dreams in medical illness.

The following articles deal with dreams and depression. Greenberg, R., and C. Pearlman, et al. "Depression: variability of intrapsychic and sleep parameters." *J. Am. Ac. Psychoanal.* 1990; 18(2):233–246. Hauri, P. "Dreams in patients remitted from reactive depression." *J. Abnorm. Psychol.* 1976; 85:1–10.

For discussion of nightmares, see Hartmann, E. *The Nightmare.* (New York: Basic Books, 1984.) Hartmann, E., et al. "Who has Nightmares? The personality of the lifelong nightmare sufferer." *Arch. Gen. Psychiatr.* 1987; 44:49–56. Kales, A., et al. "Nightmares: clinical characteristics and personality patterns." *Am. J. Psychiatr.* 1980; 137:1197–1201. Berquier, A., and R. Ashton. "Characteristics of the frequent nightmare sufferer." *J. Abnorm. Psychol.* 1992; 101(2):246–250; and Wood, J. M., et al. "Effects of the 1989 San Francisco earthquake on frequency and content of nightmares." *J. Abnorm. Psychol.* 1992; 101(2):219–224.

Lucid dreaming is covered in LaBerge, S. *Lucid Dreaming.* (New York: Ballantine Books, 1985), an entire volume dedicated to the topic. See also Gackenbach, J. "Lucid Dreaming: Individual differences in personal characteristics." *Sleep Res.* 1981; 10:145–146.

For examples of dream analysis theories of the various schools of dream theory, see Fosshage, J. L., and C. A. Loew, eds. *Dream Interpretation: A Comparative Study.* (New York: PMA Pub., 1987.)

For the phenomenological approach, see Boss, M. *The Analysis of Dreams.* (London: Rider, 1957.) Globus, G. G. *Dream Life, Wake Life: The Human Condition Through Dreams.* (Albany: State University of New York Press, 1987); and Gabel, S. "The phenomenology of the self and its objects in waking and dreaming. . . ." *J. Am. Ac. Psychoanal.* 1993; 21(3):339–362.

Chapter 19

Isakower, O. "A contribution to the patho-psychology associated with falling asleep." *Int. J. Psychoanal.* 1938; 19:331–345.

Nininger, J. collected this mass of material from patients on his wards at the Payne Whitney Psychiatric Institute, New York Hospital.

Rosen, J., et al. "Sleep disturbances in survivors of the Nazi holocaust." *Am. J. Psychiatr.* 1991; 148(1):62–66.

For two major articles on the relationship between antidepressant use and bone formation, see Faragalla, F. F., and F. F. Flach. "Studies of mineral metabolism in mental depression." *J. Nerv. Ment. Dis.* 1970; 151:120–129. Mornstad, H., et al. "Acute effects of some different anti-depressant drugs on saliva composition." *Neuropsychobiol.* 1986; 15 (2):73–79.

Chapter 20

"ABC of sleep disorders." *BMJ* 1993; 306(6892):1604–1607. Summary of prevalance of insomnia and its costs. See also Fritz, R. *Sleep Disorders: America's Hidden Nightmare.* (Napierville, Ill.: National Sleep Alert, 1993) and Leger, D. "The cost of sleep-related accidents: A report for the National Commission on Sleep Disorders Research." *Sleep* 1994; 17:84–93.

For the relationship between sleep extent and mortality, see Wingard, D. L., and L. F. Berkman, "Mortality risk associated with sleeping patterns among adults." *Sleep* 1983; 6:102–107. Kripkie, D. F., et al. "Short and long sleep and sleeping pills: Is increased mortality associated?" *Arch. Gen. Psychiatr.* 1979; 36:103–116.

For correlations between mortality times and sleep times see Mitler, M. M., et al. "Sleep, catastrophes and public policy." *Sleep* 1988; 11:100–109. Mitler, M. M. "Two-Peak 24-hour patterns in sleep, mortality, and error." *Sleep Res.* 1990; 19:399.

A basic comprehensive reference on the relationship between sleep and exercise is to be found in Shapiro, C. M. "Sleep and exercise." *Acta Physio. Scand. Suppl.* 1988; 133(574):3–54.

For the personality characteristics of persons with insomnia, see Coursey, R., M. Buchsbaum, and B. Frankel. "Personality measures and evoked responses in chronic insomniacs." *J. Abnorm. Psychol.* 1975; 84:239–249. Zorich, F. J., T. Roth, et al. "Evaluation and diagnosis of persistent insomnia." *Am. J. Psychiatr.* 1981; 138:769–773. Kales, A., et al. "Biopsychobehavioral correlates of insomnia III." *Int. J. Neurosci.* 1984; 23:43–55. Kales, A., et al. "Biopsychobehavioral correlates of insomnia V, Clinical characteristics and behavioral correlates." *Am. J. Psychiatr.* 1984; 141:1371–1376. Tan, T. L., J. D. Kales, A. Kales, et al. "Biopsychobehavioral correlates of insomnia IV: diagnosis based on DSM-111." *Am. J. Psychiatr.* 1984; 141:357–362. Hauri, P. "A cluster analysis of insomnia." *Sleep* 1983; 6(4):326–338.

For differences between good and poor sleepers see Monroe, L. J. "Psychological and physiological differences between good and poor sleepers." *J. Abnorm. Psychol.* 1967; 72:255–264. Mendelson, W. B., et al. "The experience of insomnia and daytime and nighttime functioning." *Psychiatr. Res.* 1984; 12:235–250.

For the characteristics of good and poor sleepers during the day see Marchini, E. J., et al. "What do insomniacs do, think, and feel during the day? A preliminary study." *Sleep* 1983; 6(2):147–155. Sloan, K. A., and A. D. Bertelson. "Thoughts, moods, and the daytime activities of insomniacs and good sleepers." *Sleep Res.* 1989; 16:289.

Index